Advance praise for *The Plant-Based Power Diet*

"*The Plant-Based Power Diet* presents a powerful, scientifically based program for trimming down and getting healthy. Its step-by-step approach makes changing the menu incredibly easy, and the delicious recipes will make you wish you'd tried this years ago. This book will change your life."

—Neal Barnard, M.D., president,
Physicians Committee for Responsible Medicine

"I truly believe that a plant-based, whole foods diet is the future, necessary for peak personal and environmental health. *The Plant-Based Power Diet* will help you get there."

—Brendan Brazier, bestselling author of
The Thrive Diet and formulator of Vega

"*The Plant-Based Power Diet* offers a wonderfully sensible, smart, and enthusiastic path to eating healthy—it's an excellent book for people who are new to the concept and for people who've been plant-strong for years. Highly recommended!"

—Gene Stone, author of *Forks Over Knives* and
The Secrets of People Who Never Get Sick

"If you want to pursue a vegetarian diet, Leslie Beck has created the quintessential plan of action with her book *The Plant-Based Power Diet*. This book outlines everything you need to know on how to get your protein, calcium, iron and omega-3 needs met to ensure vibrant health. Leslie's book does good for your body, for the planet and for the future of food!"

—Julie Daniluk, R.H.N., bestselling author of
Meals That Heal Inflammation

PENGUIN

THE PLANT-BASED POWER DIET

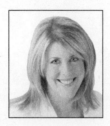

LESLIE BECK, a registered dietitian, is a leading Canadian nutritionist and the bestselling author of 12 nutrition books. Leslie writes a weekly nutrition column in *The Globe and Mail*, is a regular guest expert on CTV News Channel and can be heard one morning a week on CJAD Radio's *The Andrew Carter Morning Show* in Montreal.

Leslie has worked with many of Canada's leading businesses and international food companies and is the National Director of Nutrition for BodyScience Medical, based in Toronto, where she oversees the delivery of all nutrition and weight-management programs and works one-on-one with clients. She also regularly delivers nutrition workshops to corporate groups across North America.

Visit Leslie's website at www.lesliebeck.com.

ALSO BY LESLIE BECK

LESLIE BECK RD

THE PLANT-BASED
POWER
DIET

10 Simple Steps to
a Healthier, Leaner,
Energetic You

PENGUIN
an imprint of Penguin Canada

Published by the Penguin Group
Penguin Group (Canada), 90 Eglinton Avenue East, Suite 700, Toronto, Ontario, Canada M4P 2Y3

Penguin Group (USA) Inc., 375 Hudson Street, New York, New York 10014, U.S.A.
Penguin Books Ltd, 80 Strand, London WC2R 0RL, England
Penguin Ireland, 25 St Stephen's Green, Dublin 2, Ireland (a division of Penguin Books Ltd)
Penguin Group (Australia), 707 Collins Street, Melbourne, Victoria 3008, Australia
(a division of Pearson Australia Group Pty Ltd)
Penguin Books India Pvt Ltd, 11 Community Centre, Panchsheel Park, New Delhi – 110 017, India
Penguin Group (NZ), 67 Apollo Drive, Rosedale, Auckland 0632, New Zealand
(a division of Pearson New Zealand Ltd)
Penguin Books (South Africa) (Pty) Ltd, 24 Sturdee Avenue, Rosebank, Johannesburg 2196, South Africa

Penguin Books Ltd, Registered Offices: 80 Strand, London WC2R 0RL, England

First published 2013

1 2 3 4 5 6 7 8 9 10 (WEB)

Manufactured in Canada.

LIBRARY AND ARCHIVES CANADA CATALOGUING IN PUBLICATION

Beck, Leslie (Leslie C.)
The plant-based power diet : 10 simple steps to a healthier, leaner, energetic you / Leslie Beck.

Includes index.

ISBN 978-0-14-318387-7

1. Vegetarianism. 2. Vegetarian cooking. I. Title.

TX392.B43 2013   613.2'62   C2012-906278-2

Visit the Penguin Canada website at **www.penguin.ca**

Special and corporate bulk purchase rates available; please see **www.penguin.ca/corporatesales** or call 1-800-810-3104, ext. 2477.

ALWAYS LEARNING   **PEARSON**

Contents

Introduction   ix

Part 1 A Plant-Based Diet in 10 Simple Steps   1

Step 1   Optimize Your Health with Plant-Based Eating   2
Step 2   Learn Why a Plant-Based Diet Makes So Much Sense   11
Step 3   Become Familiar with Whole Foods, Plant-Based Eating   23
Step 4   Get All of Your Protein from Plant Sources   60
Step 5   Know Your Carbohydrates: Grains, Gluten and More   74
Step 6   Include the Right Balance of Healthy Fats   87
Step 7   Find Your Calcium in Non-Dairy Sources   98
Step 8   Maximize Your Nutrients with a Wide Mix of Plant Foods   109
Step 9   Transition to *The Plant-Based Power Diet*   125
Step 10 Stock Your Plant-Based Pantry   131

Part 2 The Plant-Based Power Diet   141

The Plant-Based Power Diet Food Groups and Serving Sizes   142
The Plant-Based Power Diet Meal Plans   149
The Plant-Based Power Diet 7-Day Menu Plan   154

Part 3 The Plant-Based Power Diet Recipes   163

References   217
Index   220

Introduction

While we don't have statistics, more and more Canadians are interested in plant-based eating. As a dietitian in private practice, my clients often ask me to design meal plans that contain little or no animal foods. People want to be healthy—and stay healthy longer—and are turning to food to help them do just that. There's solid evidence that plant-based diets have substantial health benefits, from preventing heart disease, diabetes and certain cancers to halting disease progression in its tracks. In fact, President Bill Clinton brought international attention to plant-based eating after crediting his weight loss and improved health to a vegan diet. Many professional athletes have also turned to a plant-based diet to give themselves a competitive edge.

There's more than presidential and celebrity endorsements to the growing popularity of plant-based eating. Today, it's easier to go meat- and dairy-free. No longer do you have to go to your local health food store to seek out plant-based alternatives. You'll find an enormous selection of plant foods—from non-dairy milks to meat substitutes to vegan food products—in mainstream grocery stores. When it comes to grains, we've never had more choice: quinoa, millet and farro, to name just a few. And judging by the number of plant-based cookbooks available, it seems that people are very interested in cooking plant-based meals.

There are plenty of good reasons to adopt a plant-based diet. We live in a society in which being overweight is considered the norm, not the exception, and in which type 2 diabetes is now an epidemic. Even with powerful drugs that lower cholesterol and blood pressure, heart disease continues to kill us. Its early signs are even showing up in kids. And a growing number of cancers are being clearly linked to diet and obesity. The good news is that the majority of chronic illnesses that afflict us today are largely preventable with a plant-based diet.

It is entirely possible to avoid diabetes, ward off a heart attack and drastically lower your chance of developing many cancers by changing your diet. It's as simple as that. A plant-based diet has enormous potential to optimize your health, restore your energy and rid your body of excess fat. It's an evidence-based approach to eating that's clean, kind to animals and easy on the environment. And it offers more fibre, antioxidants and health-enhancing phytochemicals than any other diet.

Whether this is your first venture into the world of plant-based eating or you're already dabbling in it, *The Plant-Based Power Diet* shows you, step by step, how to follow the principles of plant-based nutrition and get all the nutrients you need. Each and every step of *The Plant-Based Power Diet* is designed to help you maximize your nutrition by eating a mix of nutritious, whole foods. You'll learn quick and easy ways to incorporate a wide variety of vegetables, fruits, legumes and whole grains into your daily diet to boost your intake of fibre, vitamins, minerals and antioxidants. In the process, you'll discover new and delicious foods that will become staples in your diet.

WHAT'S INSIDE *THE PLANT-BASED POWER DIET*
This book is divided into three parts, each of which gives you valuable information, tips and tools to help you adopt a 100 percent plant-based diet. In Part 1, A Plant-Based Diet in 10 Simple Steps, you'll find everything you need to know about moving from a diet based on animal foods to one centred on plants. You'll learn the incredible health benefits of plant-based eating and why such a diet is better for the environment and compassionate to animals. I outline a way of eating that's based on five new food groups along with plenty of tips for choosing some of the most nutritious foods on the planet, including legumes, whole grains, fruit, vegetables

and healthy fats. And I show you how it's entirely possible to get all of the protein, calcium, iron and zinc your body needs from a diet that doesn't include meat and dairy.

In Part 1, you'll also find easy, practical tips to help you transition from your current diet to *The Plant-Based Power Diet*. Whether it takes you days or weeks, I offer plenty of ways to make the transition a smooth one. I also give you a list of foods and condiments that should always be in your plant-based kitchen to help you prepare a healthy, great-tasting meal in a hurry.

Part 2, *The Plant-Based Power Diet*, puts your new-found knowledge into action. There, I outline *The Plant-Based Power Diet* food groups and serving sizes. You'll find four meal plans, each one specifying a daily calorie level: 1400, 1600, 1900 or 2200 calories. Which meal plan you choose to follow will depend on your gender, activity level and weight goal. Each meal plan comes with advice to ensure that you get sufficient vitamin B_{12}, calcium, iron and omega-3 fatty acids. To help you get started, you'll also find a 7-day menu plan that includes many delicious plant-based recipes.

45 PLANT-BASED RECIPES TO GET YOU STARTED
In Part 3, you'll find 45 delicious recipes to get you started on the path to plant-based eating—and to a healthier, leaner and happier you. Each recipe is accompanied by an analysis that provides the calorie, protein, fat, carbohydrate, fibre, cholesterol and sodium content per serving. Whether you use these recipes by following the 7-day menu plan or try them one by one, I hope that many will become staple dishes in your plant-based lifestyle.

So let's get started. It's time to become immersed in the world of plant-based nutrition. It's a way of eating that has the potential to offer enormous health benefits, not to mention add a variety of delicious and nutrient-rich foods to your diet. Enjoy the path to plant-based eating.

Leslie Beck, RD
Toronto, 2013

PART 1
A Plant-Based Diet in 10 Simple Steps

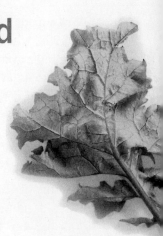

Step 1

Optimize Your Health with Plant-Based Eating

We've made remarkable strides in medicine over the past century. In 1900, when tuberculosis and pneumonia were leading causes of death, the average life expectancy was age 48. Today Canadians are living to an average age of 81, thanks to improvements in sanitation, food and water and the advent of vaccines and antibiotics. Greater access to health care, earlier detection of chronic diseases and advances in medicine are helping us live longer than we did even a decade ago.

We're also keenly interested in living a longer, healthy life. The majority of Canadians—85 percent—consider nutrition important when deciding what to eat. It's pretty hard not to be aware of the link between food and health. We're bombarded every day with healthy-living messages from the media, the Internet, health experts, friends and family. Books on health and diet dominate bestseller lists. Labels on food packages broadcast countless health claims. Reality TV shows showcasing the extreme efforts of very overweight people to achieve dramatic—and unsafe—weight loss are watched by millions.

Despite the fact that nutrition information is everywhere, many of us continue to eat too many calories and too much artery-clogging fat, sodium and sugar. We're eating too much of the wrong food and not nearly enough of the right food. We're an overfed and undernourished bunch. Most North Americans eat animal foods at every meal, 7 days a week, 365 days a year. Most civilizations have included some meat in their diet since prehistoric times. After World War II, meat and dairy became mass-produced, allowing millions of people to afford them. As animal foods become a constant fixture on our menu, we began to experience health problems—obesity, gout, heart disease, diabetes and so on—that had previously afflicted only the rich, who could afford these foods.

Our Western dietary ways—characterized by meat, dairy and processed foods—have infiltrated countries where people historically ate a plant-based diet and food-related health problems were virtually non-existent. People living in China, Japan, India, parts of Africa and other countries now share our penchant for meat, fast food and processed foods. In these countries, where McDonald's Big Macs are popular with adults and kids, more and more people are becoming overweight and developing heart disease, diabetes and cancer. In fact, worldwide obesity has more than doubled since 1980. Our Western diet—here and around the world—is paving the way for poor health. In fact, we are likely eating our way to an early grave.

Today's top killers are no longer infectious diseases. They're chronic diseases that progress slowly and last a long time. Chronic diseases such as heart disease, diabetes and cancer are among the leading causes of death in the world. In North America, billions of dollars are spent every year to treat people who suffer from a chronic disease. Yet many of these diseases can be avoided by making smart lifestyle choices. Experts estimate that controlling weight, eating a healthy diet, exercising and not smoking would prevent 8 out of 10 cases of heart disease and half of all cancers. Adopting those healthy habits would also avert 9 out of 10 cases of type 2 diabetes. Think about that for a moment. Type 2 diabetes, which is a significant risk factor for heart attack, is largely preventable. Yet we're witnessing an epidemic of it in this country. As you'll learn, switching to a plant-based diet is a powerful way to reduce your risk for many different chronic diseases.

CARDIOVASCULAR DISEASE

Coronary heart disease (heart disease) and stroke are forms of cardiovascular disease, conditions caused by hardening and narrowing of the arteries (atherosclerosis). Together, they are the second leading cause of death in Canada, accounting for 29 percent of all deaths.[1] (As you'll soon read, cancer is now our number one killer.)

Heart disease, which accounts for 54 percent of all cardio-vascular deaths, develops when fatty materials, calcium and plaques build up in arteries that supply blood to the heart. This buildup narrows the arteries and prevents the heart from getting enough blood, potentially leading to a heart attack. In Canada, a heart attack occurs every seven minutes.

By definition, a stroke is a sudden loss of brain function. The majority of strokes—80 percent—are called ischemic strokes. They're caused by an interruption of blood flow to the brain due to a blood clot, causing brain cells in the affected area to die. Like heart disease, a buildup of plaques in the arteries is involved in most ischemic strokes. In this case, however, these plaques narrow the arteries that deliver blood to the brain.

Nine in 10 Canadians have at least one modifiable risk factor for heart disease and stroke—that is, risk factors that can be prevented or controlled by adjusting lifestyle habits.

Risk Factors for Heart Disease and Stroke
- Diabetes
- High blood cholesterol
- High blood pressure
- Being overweight
- Excessive alcohol consumption
- Sedentary lifestyle
- Smoking
- Stress

Animal foods like meat and dairy contain saturated fat and cholesterol, substances that promote the accumulation of fatty plaques in artery walls. Plant-based foods, on the other hand, are void of artery-clogging fat. And they contain hundreds of protective compounds that work to keep blood vessels healthy and relaxed.

That's not all: Groundbreaking research has proven that a plant-based diet can reverse the progression of heart disease.

DIABETES

Diabetes is growing at epidemic levels across the country. Today, one in four Canadians (9 million) has diabetes or pre-diabetes, and if the trend continues, this number is expected to rise to one in three by 2020.[2] What's to blame for this? Certainly, an aging population, but that's not all. A diet that contributes to being overweight and our sedentary lifestyle are key culprits.

Type 2 diabetes, which accounts for 90 percent of all cases of the disease, is fuelling this epidemic. The condition occurs when the pancreas does not produce enough insulin—the hormone that clears sugar (glucose) from the bloodstream—or when the body's cells can't use insulin properly. As a result, a high level of glucose circulates in the bloodstream and, if left untreated, causes damage to blood vessels, tissues and organs. Diabetes is serious business. It can lead to heart disease, kidney disease, eye disease, erectile dysfunction and nerve damage.

Pre-diabetes, also called impaired fasting glucose, is diagnosed when your fasting blood glucose reading is higher than normal (a normal fasting glucose is 4 to 6 mmol/L) but not high enough to be considered type 2 diabetes. (A diagnosis of type 2 diabetes requires a fasting blood glucose of 7 mmol/L or higher.) That doesn't mean that a slightly elevated blood sugar isn't dangerous. Quite the contrary. Studies show that some of the long-term complications of diabetes—heart disease and nerve damage—can begin during pre-diabetes. While not everyone with pre-diabetes will develop full-blown type 2 diabetes, many people will.

The risk of type 2 diabetes increases as you get older, especially after age 40. That's probably because as we age we tend to gain weight and lose muscle. But the disease is being diagnosed in children and teenagers, something unheard of 40 years ago. In fact, type 2 diabetes used to be called adult-onset diabetes. The name was changed when the disease started showing up in young people. It turns out that there are risk factors more important than age that contribute to the development of type 2 diabetes. And as you'll see, many of them can be eradicated by making changes to your diet.

Risk Factors for Type 2 Diabetes
• Pre-diabetes
• Family history: having a parent or sibling with type 2 diabetes
• Heart disease
• High blood cholesterol
• High blood pressure
• Being overweight, especially around your abdomen
• History of gestational diabetes (diabetes during pregnancy)

Adopting a plant-based diet has been shown to outperform a diet based on animal foods in helping people with diabetes to manage their condition. In fact, this diet is so effective that it's helped people achieve normal, non-diabetic blood-sugar readings.

OBESITY
Like the many chronic diseases to which it's linked, obesity is also on the rise in Canada. Today, one in four Canadian adults is obese. So are 12 percent of young people aged 5 to 17.[3] What's more, obesity rates have doubled among adults and youth over the past 30 years. That's alarming since being obese increases the likelihood that you'll develop health problems, many of them serious and life threatening. Heart disease, stroke, high blood pressure, type 2 diabetes, certain cancers, osteoarthritis and sleep apnea are all related to being overweight or obese.

If your body mass index (BMI) is 30 or greater, you're considered obese. BMI is calculated as your weight in kilograms divided by the square of your height in metres. If you don't know your BMI, you can find many BMI calculators online. For most people, having a BMI of 30 means being about 30 pounds (14 kilograms) overweight. Having a BMI between 25 and 29.9 is classified as overweight.

Experts blame the "obesogenic" environment in which we live for our expanding national waistline. We rely on cars to take us— and our kids—everywhere. Many of us live in suburbs so spread out that biking or walking to work, school or the grocery store isn't an option. In our modern world, highly processed and fast foods are more accessible than fresh produce and whole grains. The bottom line: We live in an environment that encourages us to eat and drink more calories than we burn off.

Even if you do live in an obesogenic neighbourhood, obesity is not inevitable. Adopting a plant-based diet can help you achieve and maintain a healthy and lean body weight.

CANCER

Cancer is now the leading cause of death in Canada, overtaking cardiovascular disease, which until recently had long been our number one killer. It's estimated that roughly one-third of all cancer deaths are due to dietary factors alone. Furthermore, experts believe that as much as 80 percent of breast, colorectal and prostate cancers—three of the most commonly diagnosed cancers—is caused by diet.[4]

Simply put, cancer is a disease in which abnormal cells grow out of control. When enough of these cells accumulate, a tumour forms. Finally, if the cancer cells are able to break away from the tumour, they can circulate through the body and take up residence in another organ, a process called metastasis. Cancer is the result of an interaction between genes and environmental factors. In other words, even if you are predisposed to cancer because you have a faulty gene, you may never develop the disease if you eat a healthy diet packed with disease-fighting nutrient- and antioxidant-rich foods.

The link between cancer and diet is not new. We've known for years that people who eat too much fatty food, especially meat, and too few plant foods such as grains, fruits and vegetables and legumes, have a higher cancer risk. The foods we eat—and don't eat—affect hormones in the body and our immune system. While animal foods contain potentially cancer-causing compounds, plant foods provide vitamins, minerals, antioxidants and phytochemicals that can protect the body. (Phytochemicals are naturally occurring compounds found in plant foods that work in many different ways to fight disease.)

Being overweight also increases the risk of certain cancers. There's convincing evidence that carrying excess body fat increases the risk of colorectal, breast (in post-menopausal women), endometrium, esophagus, pancreas, thyroid, gallbladder and kidney cancers. Obesity may increase cancer risk in a number of ways. Fat cells produce certain hormones, such as estrogen, that may trigger tumour growth. People who are obese often have elevated levels of insulin and insulin-like growth factors that could promote the growth of certain cancers. As well, obesity is associated with low-grade inflammation in the body, which has been linked to an increased cancer risk.

The good news is that a plant-based diet guards against cancer on a number of fronts. It supplies your body with a plethora of cancer-fighting nutrients and phytochemicals. Its lower calorie content—compared to a diet based on meat and dairy—helps keep you slim. And a plant-based diet also contains many different anti-inflammatory compounds, which reduce and prevent inflammation in the body.

OSTEOPOROSIS

Many people don't give osteoporosis much thought. Too often it's viewed as a disease that frail elderly people get. While the disease mainly strikes people over 50, it can occur at any age. And it's more common than you might think. At least one in three women and one in five men will suffer from a bone fracture caused by osteoporosis in their lifetime.[5] You may not realize that osteoporotic bone fractures are more common than heart attack, stroke and breast cancer combined. Or that a woman's lifetime risk of hip fracture is greater than her lifetime risk of developing breast cancer.

A hip fracture caused by osteoporosis may not sound as life threatening as a heart attack, but it is. Thirty percent of people who suffer a hip fracture will die of complications from it—23 percent of them within a year. I witnessed this first-hand after my grandmother fell and broke her hip. She died in hospital within a week.

Osteoporosis is a disease that causes bones to become weak and brittle, increasing the risk of fracture. Risk factors include being age

65 or older, suffering a fracture after age 40, a family history of hip fracture, early menopause, having a medical condition that reduces the absorption of vitamins and minerals (e.g., celiac disease, Crohn's disease) and long-term use of medications called corticosteroids (e.g., prednisone).

When it comes to your diet, getting too little calcium and vitamin D and consuming too many soft drinks and excess caffeine and alcohol also increase the risk. So does a diet that's heavy on animal protein. Diets high in meat and dairy cause the kidneys to excrete calcium and have been linked to a greater risk of fractures.

Plant foods deliver an abundance of nutrients that are needed to keep bones strong as we age. Calcium and vitamin K in leafy green vegetables, magnesium in beans, lentils and nuts, and phytochemicals in soy foods all play a role in the prevention of osteoporosis.

ALZHEIMER'S DISEASE

As baby boomers age, an increasing number of Canadians will develop Alzheimer's disease. In 2008, one person was diagnosed with the disease every five minutes. Within a generation, it's expected that one person will be diagnosed every two minutes. By 2038, the number of Canadians living with Alzheimer's disease will more than double, skyrocketing to 1 125 200.[6]

Alzheimer's disease is a relentless, fatal disease that kills brain cells. It's the most common cause of dementia, accounting for nearly two-thirds of cases. Like heart disease, diabetes and other chronic diseases, it is not a normal part of aging. Some risk factors, such as age and genetics, you can't do anything about. But others you can. For instance, high cholesterol, high blood pressure, obesity and type 2 diabetes—all of which are risk factors for heart disease and stroke—are also risk factors for Alzheimer's disease. The more unlikely you are to be healthy, the more likely you are to get the disease.

It makes sense, then, that the same diet strategies that protect your arteries and keep you lean can guard against Alzheimer's disease. Studies have clearly demonstrated that a diet low in saturated fat (a.k.a. animal fat) is protective. What's more, people who eat higher amounts of plant foods rich in vitamin E, vitamin C, beta-carotene and numerous phytochemicals are less likely to develop Alzheimer's disease.

PREVENTING ILLNESS—AND OPTIMIZING HEALTH— WITH *THE PLANT-BASED POWER DIET*

There's overwhelming evidence that a diet based on plant foods filled with nutrients, antioxidants and disease-fighting phyto-chemicals can prevent—and even reverse—many chronic diseases. Researchers and doctors believe that the higher the percentage of one's diet that comes from whole plant foods, the lower one's risk of chronic disease. In other words, you'll get better results health-wise if you eat *only* plant-based foods. Experts in the field of plant-based nutrition believe that achieving optimum health requires eating a diet that's free of animal foods—no meat, chicken, fish, eggs or dairy.

Many people find it easy to go meat- and dairy-free and will jump right into my *Plant-Based Power Diet*. But others find it more challenging to abandon animal foods "cold turkey," so to speak. The good news is that you don't have to change your diet overnight. I'll give you plenty of tips and tools to gradually transition to a plant-based diet. A step-by-step guide will help you add more plant foods to your meals every day. Once you savour new tastes and experi-ence the new-found energy that comes from eating plant-based meals, it will be only a matter of time before you take the plunge into the world of plant-based nutrition. And as you'll read in the next chapter, there are reasons beyond health that support eating a diet built solely on plant foods.

Learn Why a Plant-Based Diet Makes So Much Sense

People choose foods to eat based on many things: taste, convenience, advertising, price and nutrition are all factors. For many people, realizing a certain health benefit matters most when deciding what to eat. Others make dietary decisions based on environmental and moral considerations.

A plant-based diet appeals to people for many reasons. It's undeniably good for your health and has the potential to stave off heart disease, stroke, type 2 diabetes, obesity and many other chronic diseases. Those are powerful reasons to adopt such a diet, but there are other reasons as well. You may not realize that raising livestock for meat generates more greenhouse gas emissions than driving cars. It's also a major contributor to land and water degradation. And a plant-based diet is one that is much kinder to animals.

EXCEPTIONALLY GOOD FOR YOUR HEALTH

There's convincing evidence that a plant-based diet is clearly associated with many health advantages. Studies have consistently found that people who eat a plant-based diet have a much lower risk of coronary heart disease than meat eaters. Researchers attribute this to the favourable effect of a plant-based diet on many risk factors for heart disease. Plant-based eaters have lower cholesterol and blood pressure levels than do people who regularly eat animal foods.[1,2]

Non–meat eaters also have a lower risk of metabolic syndrome, a cluster of risk factors that doubles the risk of heart attack and increases the likelihood of developing type 2 diabetes fivefold. A person is thought to have metabolic syndrome if he or she has a large waist circumference plus two or more of the following: high blood triglycerides (blood fats), high blood pressure, elevated fasting blood sugar and low HDL (good) cholesterol. Plant-based eaters have lower triglyceride and fasting blood sugar levels, lower blood pressure and, not surprisingly, a smaller waist size than meat eaters.[3]

Plant-based diet in action: reversing heart disease

Dr. Caldwell B. Esselstyn Jr. was a surgeon, clinician and researcher at the prestigious Cleveland Clinic for 35 years. Today he runs the cardiovascular and reversal program at the Cleveland Clinic's Wellness Institute. His research provides convincing evidence that a low-fat, plant-based diet can not only stop the progression of heart disease, but also reverse its effects. Based on the observation that wherever people around the globe ate a plant-based diet cardiovascular disease was rare, he embarked on his own 20-year study to treat heart disease.

Dr. Esselstyn enrolled 24 patients with severe progressive coronary heart disease, who were basically told by their cardiologists that they had a very poor outlook. The goal was to use a plant-based diet to reduce patients' total cholesterol levels to less than 3.88 mmol/L (150 mg/dL), the level seen in cultures where heart disease is virtually non-existent. The plan was to see what effect this low cholesterol level had on the health of their hearts.

Eighteen patients stuck with the diet program. Every one of these volunteers achieved the blood cholesterol target. Angiograms—special x-rays of the coronary arteries—demonstrated that sustaining low blood cholesterol levels eliminated progression of heart disease. The flow of blood through the coronary arteries to the heart improved, and in many patients these arteries were measurably wider. People who entered the study with angina—chest pain caused by an inadequate blood supply to the heart—saw their pain disappear or greatly improve. Exercise capacity also improved.[4] Two decades later, Dr. Esselstyn's patients continue to follow his plant-based diet and remain symptom-free.

People who follow a plant-based diet also have half the risk of developing type 2 diabetes as meat eaters. And they're less likely to be overweight. Studies show that the more closely a person adheres to a 100 percent plant-based diet, the lower—and healthier—their body weight is.[5,6] A plant-based diet also guards against cancer.

Plant-based diet in action: reversing diabetes

Dr. Neal Barnard is a professor of medicine at the George Washington University School of Medicine and Health Sciences and president of the non-profit Physicians Committee for Responsible Medicine. In a series of studies, he has proven that an entirely plant-based diet can cut blood sugar, improve insulin sensitivity (the body's ability to respond to insulin) and reduce or eliminate the need for medications in people with type 2 diabetes. And unlike medications, the diet's side effects were positive: weight loss, lower cholesterol levels, lower blood pressure and increased energy.

Dr. Barnard's most recent research study compared the effectiveness of a low-fat, plant-based diet with the American Diabetes Association (ADA) diet in 99 people with type 2 diabetes. The plant-based diet outperformed the previous gold standard diet: it controlled blood sugar three times more effectively. It also resulted in more weight loss and better cholesterol levels than the ADA diet.[7] What's more, the study's volunteers preferred the plant-based diet to the standard diabetic diet!

A plant-based diet is a powerful way to boost insulin sensitivity and bring blood sugar under control. It can also reverse the decline in health experienced by many people with diabetes: increasing weight, slowly rising blood sugar and worsening complications. Following a plant-based diet may even help you drive your blood sugar down to a non-diabetic level. Keep in mind, however, that a person's genetic predisposition to type 2 diabetes will not go away. However, consistently following a plant-based diet can help ensure that your blood sugar doesn't swing into the diabetic range ever again.

Researchers have observed that, compared to non-vegetarians, vegetarians have lower cancer rates, especially for colorectal cancer. (Eating red meat and processed meat frequently is a clear risk factor for colorectal cancer.)

If a plant-based diet can ward off high blood pressure, high cholesterol, heart disease, diabetes, obesity and certain cancers, can it help you live longer? According to researchers, the answer is yes. Data from North America and Europe suggest that a diet that includes very little meat can add almost four years to your life.[8] And research from the United Kingdom revealed that, compared to national rates, vegetarians are much less likely to die from any of these causes, especially from coronary heart disease.[9]

How a Plant-Based Diet Keeps You Healthy

There are many ways in which a plant-based diet can keep you exceptionally healthy. Unlike animal foods, fruit, vegetables, legumes, nuts and whole grains don't contain saturated fat or cholesterol, so they help keep your blood cholesterol at a healthy level. Saturated fat can also impair your body's ability to properly use insulin, the hormone that clears sugar from the bloodstream. Plant foods are also naturally low in sodium.

The health benefits of a plant-based diet aren't attributed only to the fact that these foods lack unhealthy ingredients found in animal foods. Perhaps more importantly, plant foods also deliver a wealth of health-promoting compounds, many of which don't exist in animal foods. Plant foods contain thousands of phytochemicals (*phyto* means "plant" in Greek), natural compounds found in fruit, vegetables, beans, nuts, grains, herbs, tea leaves and other plant foods. By closely studying phytochemicals, scientists have learned that they perform many actions in the body to fend off disease.

THE DISEASE-FIGHTING POWER OF PHYTOCHEMICALS

Many phytochemicals—along with certain vitamins and minerals— act as antioxidants neutralizing dangerous free radicals before they can harm cells. Free radicals are unstable oxygen molecules that your body produces normally during its metabolic processes. They're also generated by cigarette smoking, drinking excess alcohol, eating a diet high in saturated fat and exposure to air pollution. A heavy free radical load can overwhelm your body's ability to destroy them, creating a state called oxidative stress. Oxidative stress has been implicated as a cause of many health problems, including athero-sclerosis, heart attack, cancer, Alzheimer's disease, arthritis, cataract and macular degeneration.

Other phytochemicals reduce inflammation in the body. Ongoing low-grade inflammation harms the body and, like oxida-tive stress, is recognized as a major determinant of many age-related diseases. A steady intake of high-fat animal foods increases the body's production of inflammatory chemicals while a plant-based diet boosts the level of anti-inflammatory compounds that are protective from disease. Many phytochemicals in fruit, vegetables, legumes, soybeans and whole grains also possess anti-cancer properties. For instance, phytochemicals called flavonoids found in berries, citrus fruit and soybeans have been shown to stop the growth of cancer cells and help the liver detoxify cancer-causing substances.

Some phytochemicals have hormone-like actions that are believed to help defend against certain cancers. For example, phytochemicals in soybeans called isoflavones can bind to estrogen receptors on breast cells. By doing so, isoflavones block the ability of a woman's own estrogen to take that spot. Studies suggest that by acting like weak forms of the body's own estrogen, a regular intake of soy foods could help lower the risk of breast cancer. That's because certain risk factors for breast cancer are related to the length of time breast cells are exposed to the body's own circulating estrogen. It's thought that estrogen can promote the growth of breast cancer cells. Soy isoflavones are also thought to guard against prostate cancer. There's also evidence that phytochemicals in flaxseeds, called lignans, play a role in preventing hormone-related cancers.

Fruit, vegetables, beans, lentils and nuts are excellent sources of vitamins and minerals. They're especially rich in calcium, magne-sium and potassium, minerals that keep your blood vessels relaxed.

Getting enough potassium from plant foods also allows your kidneys to excrete more sodium, which can help keep your blood pressure from rising.

Many plant foods have a low glycemic index. Foods that have a low glycemic index are digested more slowly than high glycemic foods like sugary drinks, sweets and many refined (white) starchy foods. That means your blood sugar and insulin rise gradually, rather than quickly. A low glycemic diet is linked with a lower risk of type 2 diabetes and colon and breast cancers. The list of low glycemic plant foods is long: large-flake and steel-cut oats, brown rice, quinoa, pasta, sweet potatoes, black beans, lentils, tofu, nuts, apples, berries, oranges, peaches and pears are just a few examples.

PROTECTS THE ENVIRONMENT

It wasn't long ago that our steak and eggs came from animals that grazed, often side by side, in an open pasture on a family-owned farm. But those days are gone. One of the most significant changes in North America that occurred in the past generation was the shift from small and medium-sized farms to large intensive livestock operations (ILOs). ILOs, or factory farms as they're often called, are large-scale industrial operations that house hundreds or thousands of food animals—cattle, pigs, chickens and turkeys—in extremely cramped conditions. These animals rarely, if ever, see the light of day.

In Canada, more than 700 million animals—20 times the size of the country's population—are raised each year for food on ILOs, most of which are owned and controlled by a handful of large corporations.[10] The livestock industry employs methods to produce large volumes of meat, poultry, eggs and milk as quickly and cheaply as possible. And it's done at a cost to the environment. Compared to any other human activity, animal agriculture contributes to more greenhouse gases, uses more water and more land and is an enormous threat to biodiversity (biodiversity is the number and variety of plant and animal species in a given geographical region).

The rising demand for meat around the world—global demand is expected to double by 2020—will put an incredible strain on scarce land, water and other natural resources. By eating a plant-based diet you are playing a role in preserving our precious environment.

Livestock and Climate Change

Intensive livestock operations have a heavy carbon footprint; they're huge greenhouse gas emitters. Greenhouse gases (GHGs), such as carbon dioxide, methane and nitrous oxide, trap heat in the atmosphere through a process called the greenhouse effect. The more GHGs, the more heat that gets trapped. The result is global warming, which causes climate change. Animal agriculture accounts for nearly one-fifth of the world's human-caused GHG emissions. The enormous rise in livestock production means that more carbon dioxide is emitted as animals breathe and more methane is released through natural digestive processes. Plus, the enormous quantity of urine and manure that these animals produce discharges nitrous oxide and methane into the environment.

Carbon dioxide emissions from the livestock industry also come from fossil fuel burning to produce fertilizer used to grow animal feed, to operate large machinery and to store and transport meat, eggs and milk.

Livestock and Land Degradation

It takes a lot of land to raise rib-eye steak, a heck of a lot more than is needed to grow broccoli or spinach. It's estimated that livestock production occupies one-third of the Earth's land that's suitable for growing crops. Most of this land is used to grow crops like corn, barley, canola and soy that are fed to the animals. The growth of livestock production is a major driver of global deforestation (the conversion of forest to pasture and cropland). The problem is most prominent in Latin America, where 70 percent of previously forested land is now occupied by pastures.

Raising animals for food is a very inefficient process. Animals eat large quantities of grain, corn and soybeans but they produce comparatively small quantities of meat, dairy or eggs. Did you know it can take as much as 16 pounds of grain to produce just

1 pound of meat? In fact, 70 percent of the cereal crops grown in the United States are used to feed livestock, not people.

Livestock and Water Use and Pollution

Raising livestock is a huge drain on the Earth's precious water supply, accounting for 70 percent of total global water usage. Roughly half of this water is used to grow crops to feed the animals. Large volumes of water are also needed for the billions of animals to drink and to clean out waste from barns, transport trucks and slaughterhouses. According to the World Society for the Protection of Animals, it takes 100 times more water to produce one kilogram of animal protein than it does to produce one kilogram of plant protein.[11]

The livestock industry doesn't just consume a massive quantity of water, but also pollutes it. Factory farms generate far more manure than can be properly disposed of. Some of the excess waste is stored in pits, which leak their contents into groundwater and streams. Unlike human sewage, animal waste is not treated to kill pathogens. As a result, disease-causing bacteria and viruses can seep into drinking water, harming the health of nearby residents. A prime example of this risk is the tragedy that occurred in Walkerton, Ontario, in 2000. Seven people died and more than 2300 became severely ill after drinking water contaminated with a dangerous strain of *E. coli*. The source of the contamination was cattle manure.

Industrial fertilizers and manure that are sprayed on fields also carry concentrated amounts of nitrogen and phosphorus into lakes and rivers. When these chemicals enter a waterway, they stimulate the rapid growth of toxic algae. This creates what's called an algae bloom—a thick mat of scum on the water's surface. Algae blooms are not just unsightly, but also deadly to marine life. They block much-needed sunlight from marine plants, which eventually die. Sooner or later the algae start to die and as they decay bacteria are produced that drain oxygen from the water, killing off fish and aquatic insects that need oxygen to live.

Antibiotic Resistance

Animals raised on intensive livestock operations are routinely given antibiotics to speed up their growth and prevent infectious disease that can easily arise by living in such confined quarters. Believe it or not, 70 percent of the antibiotics used in the United States are given to livestock, not people. The situation is similar in Canada, where a considerable amount of antibiotics are used to promote the growth of livestock, rather than to treat infections. What's more, antibiotics can be detected in our soil and surface waters.

The problem is that many of these drugs are similar to the ones used to treat infections in humans. The concern is that constant exposure to antibiotics could cause the proliferation of antibiotic-resistant bacteria, making diseases in people and animals more difficult to treat. That's why the European Union banned the use of antibiotics to promote growth in livestock in 2006. Both the Canadian and American Medical Associations support such a ban in North America.

Loss of Biodiversity

The term *biodiversity* refers to the variety of plant and animal life in an area. A rich biodiversity is crucial to supporting all living things: animals, fish, plants and even humans. People benefit in many ways from a diverse ecosystem. Plants absorb greenhouse gases, which can help prevent climate change. A healthy biodiversity of species also provides a variety of foods for us to eat. And don't forget that many of our prescription drugs and natural health products come from plants.

Unfortunately, we're using up natural resources before they can be renewed and the livestock industry is a major player in the reduction in biodiversity. Deforestation, land degradation, pollution, climate change and overfishing are all big threats to biodiversity.

The Impact of Fisheries

Industrial-scale fish farming also exacts an ecological toll on the marine environment. Farmed salmon, for example, are typically raised in ocean nets with thousands of fish crammed into each net.

They're fed wild fish—it takes roughly three pounds of wild fish to produce one pound of farmed fish—that can escape, sometimes carrying disease and parasites. Because farmed fish live in such confined quarters, they're given drugs and pesticides to fend off sea lice—a bane to salmon farmers—and infection. These chemicals can enter the environment, potentially harming other sea life and causing antibiotic resistance. Fish farms also generate pollution from feces and uneaten feed that leaks into the surrounding environment. Farmed fish can also escape from their net pens and spread disease to local wild fish and take over habitat from wild fish.

Open-sea fishing can also harm the environment. The impact of overfishing on the loss of certain fish species has been known for a long time. Fishing practices can also damage the sea floor, which fish depend on for their survival. Nooks, boulders and special burrows that fish create provide important hiding and feeding places for young fish and other sea animals. Bottom trawling, in which nets are dragged across the bottom of the ocean, pulls up nearly all plants, animals and rocks. Once the sea floor is damaged, it takes hundreds of years to grow back.

Bycatch also depletes ocean life. Bycatch refers to the sea life that is caught by accident while fishing for another species. Dolphins, sea turtles, seals, whales, sharks, swordfish and red snapper all are caught by accident and drown. Young fish, which could otherwise rebuild depleted populations, are also harmed by accidental kills. It's estimated that one-quarter of world catch is wasted.

KINDER TO ANIMALS

Traditionally, cattle, pigs, chickens and turkeys led a simple life. They were raised in environments that were natural to them and for which they were biologically suited. They raised their families, breathed fresh air and felt sun on their backs. Cows grazed in open pastures, pigs rooted in the dirt and chickens built nests and pecked the ground. And their owners treated them humanely. Sadly, that's not the case on ILOs, or factory farms, where animals are seen as commodities rather than as living, breathing beings. Animals raised on ILOs live lives of stress and frustration, unable to forage and explore, see the light of day and interact with other animals.

ILOs strive to maximize output while minimizing costs. That means that animals are severely crammed together in pens, in small cages or on feedlots without access to sunlight, fresh air, open pasture or exercise. Chickens are crowded into small wire cages that severely restrict them from turning around or stretching their wings. Many hens suffer from osteoporosis and broken bones due to their lack of mobility. Calves that produce veal often live their entire lives in crates so small they can't turn around, walk, play or comfortably lie down to sleep. Breeding sows are kept in individual stalls so restrictive that the animals are hurt when they try to lie down. When pigs are close to market size, they're packed into small indoor pens with little room to move. When large enough, animals are packed tightly onto trucks and transported many kilometres, in all types of weather, to the slaughterhouse.

These animals must also endure painful procedures without the use of anaesthetic. To prevent laying hens from pecking their cage mates, their beaks are trimmed with a hot blade. Turkeys have their toes partially amputated to prevent their claws getting caught in the wire mesh on the floor of their cages. Newborn male calves are castrated shortly after being taken away from their mothers and sometimes branded. Almost immediately after birth, piglets' teeth are clipped to prevent injuries to other piglets and to their mother as they fight for the best teats. These are regular practices on ILOs and they're performed without any means to prevent or relieve pain.

Most people can't tolerate cruelty to animals. Yet many of us turn a blind eye to the industrial methods—from farm to slaughter-house—that put steak, chicken, pork, eggs and milk on our table. As Michael Pollan said in his *New York Times* blog, "To peer over the increasingly high walls of our industrial animal agriculture is not only to lose your appetite but to feel revulsion and shame."[12] Adopting a plant-based diet is a vote against animal cruelty.

A diet that serves up animal foods at every meal promotes poor health, is environmentally unsustainable and neglects animal welfare. A plant-based diet, on the other hand, promotes optimal health, is environmentally friendly and is compassionate to animals. Now it's time to learn what plant-based nutrition really means.

Step 3

Become Familiar with Whole Foods, Plant-Based Eating

When people change their diet, they usually focus on the foods they can't eat. No more french fries, no more cookies, no more chocolate and so on. A plant-based diet requires a different mindset because it focuses on all the foods you *can* eat. It emphasizes foods that come from, not surprisingly, plants: fruits, vegetables, whole grains, legumes and nuts. And it includes foods that are as close to their natural form as possible. A *whole foods*, plant-based diet eliminates highly processed foods; it includes foods that retain their fibre and portfolio of beneficial nutrients and phytochemicals that are often missing from processed foods.

While white bread is a plant-based food because it's made from wheat, it's missing the fibre, B vitamins, vitamin E, magnesium and antioxidants found in 100% whole wheat bread. (Technically, 100% whole wheat bread is processed, but it's much closer to nature than bread made from refined, white flour.) Many packaged foods that line grocery store shelves contain refined flours, added sugars, processed oils and a long list of synthetic preservatives, flavour enhancers and colourings. These foods are so processed they barely resemble the whole foods that nature intended us to eat.

PLANT-BASED VERSUS VEGETARIAN
You may be thinking that a plant-based diet sounds a lot like a vegetarian diet. There are similarities, but there are also differences. A vegetarian diet does include fruits, vegetables, grains, beans, soy foods and nuts. But not all vegetarian diets avoid animal foods. In fact, vegetarianism covers a wide range of eating styles.

Types of Vegetarian Diets

- *Semi-vegetarians* don't eat red meat but still eat a little poultry, eggs, fish and seafood.
- *Pesco-vegetarians* don't eat poultry and meat but still include fish and seafood.
- *Lacto-ovo vegetarians* eat dairy (lacto) and eggs (ovo) but exclude meat, poultry and fish.
- *Lacto-vegetarians* eat dairy but not meat, poultry, fish or eggs.
- *Vegans* avoid eating all animal foods, including meat, poultry, fish, eggs, dairy and honey (vegans regard honeybees as animals).

There's another difference between plant-based and vegetarian diets. I mentioned earlier that a plant-based diet focuses on the foods you can eat. Many vegetarians, on the other hand, are mainly concerned about those foods they can't eat. Their diets are defined by what's excluded from them. Meal planning is focused on avoiding one or more types of animal foods rather than maximizing nutrient intake by eating a variety of plant-based foods. When I meet vegetarian clients in my practice, I often see this approach to eating reflected in their nutritional intake. Meals may include pasta with tomato sauce, veggie stir-fry with rice, cheese pizza, soy burgers and nut butter sandwiches. When I analyze a day's worth of their meals and snacks, I often find it's lacking in a handful of vitamins and minerals. Too often, vegetarians omit animal foods from meals but don't eat a wide enough variety of nutrient-packed plant foods.

Is There (a Little) Room for Animal Foods?

A plant-based diet is defined by what's included in it rather than what's not, which raises a question that many people ask me. Does a plant-based diet have to be meat-free? Can I still occasionally eat a burger? Can I eat eggs for breakfast or pour milk on my cereal? The answer is no. A plant-based diet doesn't include any meat, poultry, eggs or dairy products. Doctors and scientists studying plant-based diets believe you'll gain the greatest health benefits, energy and vigour by eating a diet that is 100 percent plant-based. And of course, eating this way supports the environment and the well-being of animals. If adopting a completely plant-based diet is your goal, *The Plant-Based Power Diet* will help you make the transition from your current diet.

A NEW FOOD GUIDE TO PLANT-BASED EATING

No doubt you're familiar with Canada's Food Guide, the national tool that recommends eating a certain number of servings of foods from four main food groups every day. The four food groups—Meat and Alternatives, Milk and Alternatives, Grain Products, Vegetables and Fruit—are intended to provide the nutrients your body needs to grow, repair and stay healthy. However, our national food guide wasn't designed to meet the nutrient requirements of plant-based eaters. That's why my *Plant-Based Power Diet* is based on a system developed for the sole purpose of helping you achieve optimum nutrition from the world of plant foods.

The Plant-Based Power Diet is built on five food groups—and as you can probably guess, the meat and dairy food groups are not included. The five food groups your new plant-based diet will be centred on:

- Vegetables
- Fruit
- Legumes and Soy
- Grains and Starchy Vegetables
- Healthy Fats and Oils

Let's take a closer look at each food group.

VEGETABLES

We all know that vegetables are incredibly good for us. Yet many people don't eat nearly enough of them to reap their health benefits. That will change on *The Plant-Based Power Diet!* With a little planning, it's easy to include plenty of vegetable servings in your daily diet. One vegetable serving is equivalent to 1/2 cup (125 mL) raw or cooked vegetables, 1 cup (250 mL) salad greens and 1/2 cup (125 mL) 100% vegetable juice.

Tips to Increase Your Vegetable Intake

Breakfast	Include 1 vegetable serving. (e.g., sliced tomato on whole-grain toast with tahini, a small glass of carrot or vegetable juice)
Snacks	Keep raw vegetable sticks handy for between-meal snacks. Prepare them in advance to save time during the day. Try baby carrots, red pepper sticks, broccoli florets, zucchini slices and cherry tomatoes.
Lunch	Include at least 2 vegetable servings. (e.g., tomato juice, spinach leaves in your sandwich, a handful of baby carrots, a bowl of vegetable soup, green salad)
Dinner	Include at least 2 different vegetable servings. (e.g., carrots and broccoli, mixed vegetable stir-fry, tomato sauce with spinach served over pasta)

Vegetables are among the best sources of vitamins C and K, potassium and fibre. Many also deliver a fair bit of folate—a B vitamin that keeps our DNA healthy—and calcium. Vegetables also contain hundreds and hundreds of phytochemicals that are linked to a lower risk of heart disease and cancer, better eyesight and even improved memory. While all vegetables are good for you, some deserve special attention for their outstanding contribution to good health.

Leafy Greens

Arugula ⁂ beet greens ⁂ collard greens ⁂ dandelion greens
kale ⁂ mustard greens ⁂ leaf lettuce ⁂ rapini (broccoli raab)
romaine lettuce ⁂ spinach ⁂ Swiss chard ⁂ turnip greens

Eating more leafy green vegetables is associated with protection from lung, stomach and ovarian cancers. Greens contain plenty of vitamins A and C, which help maintain healthy body tissues, especially epithelial and mucous tissues, the body's first line of defence against invading organisms and toxins. Many are also excellent sources of the B vitamin folate, a nutrient that keeps our DNA in good repair.

Leafy greens are also linked to a lower risk of cataract and macular degeneration, an eye disease that's the leading cause of blindness in older adults. Scientists attribute their eye benefits to their exceptional content of two phytochemicals called lutein and zeaxanthin. Once consumed, lutein and zeaxanthin make their way to your eye where they protect your eye's retina and lens from free-radical damage. Scientists speculate that a daily intake of 6 to 15 milligrams of lutein plus zeaxanthin is optimal for eye health. A half-cup of cooked kale supplies 12 milligrams! A half-cup of cooked spinach has 10 milligrams!

There's yet another reason to make leafy greens a regular part of *The Plant-Based Power Diet:* to protect your bones. Thanks to their sizable vitamin K content, leafy greens have been shown to help maintain bone density and lower the risk of hip fracture.

Here's how leafy greens stack up in terms of their nutrient content.

Notable Nutrients in Leafy Green Vegetables
Per 1/2 cup (125 mL) serving, cooked (unless otherwise indicated)

	Calories	Vit. A (mcg)	Vit. C (mg)	Vit. K (mcg)	Folate (mcg)
Arugula, 1 cup raw	5	25	3	22	20
Beet greens, 1 cup raw	9	127	12	161	6
Beet greens	21	291	19	368	11
Collard greens	26	408	18	442	93
Dandelion greens, 1 cup raw	26	144	20	159	16
Dandelion greens	18	275	10	108	7
Kale	19	468	28	561	9
Leaf lettuce, 1 cup raw	9	219	11	103	22
Mustard greens	11	234	19	221.5	54
Rapini	22	150	24.5	169	47
Romaine lettuce, 1 cup raw	10	172	14	61	80
Spinach, 1 cup raw	7	149	9	153	61

	Calories	Vit. A (mcg)	Vit. C (mg)	Vit. K (mcg)	Folate (mcg)
Spinach	22	498	9.3	469	139
Swiss chard	18	283	16.6	303	8
Turnip greens	15	290	21	280	90

	Calcium (mg)	Magnesium (mg)	Iron (mg)	Potassium (mg)
Arugula, 1 cup raw	34	10	0.3	78
Beet greens, 1 cup raw	47	28	1	306
Beet greens	87	52	1.5	692
Collard greens	141	20	1.2	116
Dandelion greens, 1 cup raw	109	21	1.8	231
Dandelion greens	78	13	1	129
Kale	49	12	0.6	157
Leaf lettuce, 1 cup raw	21	8	0.5	115
Mustard greens	55	11	0.6	149
Rapini	78	18	0.85	227
Romaine lettuce, 1 cup raw	20	8	0.6	146
Spinach, 1 cup raw	31	25	0.9	177
Spinach	129	83	3.4	443
Swiss chard	51	75	2	480
Turnip greens	99	16	0.6	146

Most leafy greens can be eaten fresh in salads. Greens with larger leaves, such as romaine lettuce, kale and collard greens can be wrapped around other ingredients like a tortilla. Although they're often eaten fresh, all leafy greens can be cooked using several different methods: blanching, braising, sautéing, steaming and even microwaving. Leafy greens can also be added to stir-fries, pasta sauces, stews and soups.

COOKING LEAFY GREENS

Cooking greens actually makes them more nutritious than if they are eaten raw. That's because leafy greens contain oxalates, natural compounds that bind tightly to calcium and iron. (You'll learn more about oxalates and calcium absorption in Step 7.) Cooking greens releases their minerals from oxalates, making them more available for absorption in your gastrointestinal tract. Just don't overcook your greens! Overcooking leafy greens will reduce their vitamin C and folate content, not to mention make them taste bitter.

Whichever cooking method you choose, use the liquid that's left over to make sauces or add extra flavour and nutrients to soups, stews and pasta sauces. Keep in mind that greens shrink considerably when cooked, often to less than half their volume. One pound of greens (454 g) can easily shrink to 1 to 2 cups (250 to 500 mL) once cooked. Here's a guide to cooking leafy greens:

Blanching—A method that requires greens to be plunged into boiling water briefly, then into cold water to stop the cooking process. Blanching is used to soften the texture of some greens and provide a flavour less pungent or bitter as when raw. It's also used to heighten and set colour and flavour before freezing vegetables.

A recipe may call for greens to be blanched before the main cooking method, like sautéing. Greens that benefit from blanching include kale, collard greens, mustard greens, turnip greens and rapini. More delicate greens like spinach and arugula don't need blanching.

To blanch, bring water to boil in a large pot. Add greens to boiling water and cook for 1 to 5 minutes, or until greens have wilted. Remove from the heat and drain. Allow greens to cool before squeezing moisture from them. If they're not going to be used immediately, rinse them under cold running water and squeeze out excess moisture.

Braising—A method by which leafy greens are cooked, tightly covered, in a small amount of liquid at low heat for a lengthy period of time. The long, slow cooking develops flavour and tenderizes greens by gently breaking down their fibres. Braising can be done on top of the range or in the oven. Head-type greens (kale, Swiss chard, collard greens) may benefit from being blanched for 2 minutes before being braised.

To braise, place greens in a skillet and add broth until greens are almost covered. Add onion, garlic or any of your favourite herbs and spices. Cover the skillet and cook at a simmer for 10 to 20 minutes, or until tender. You can make a sauce to serve with the greens by boiling the cooking liquid left in the pan until most of the liquid evaporates.

Sautéing—This method cooks greens quickly in a small amount of oil in a skillet or sauté pan over direct heat. Non-stick pans will require less oil than other pans. You can also sauté in vegetable broth to keep your fat intake low.

To sauté, add greens to heated oil. Other flavourings, such as garlic, onions and chili peppers, can be sautéed with the greens. Sauté for 3 to 10 minutes, stirring constantly. Remove from the pan and serve while hot.

Steaming—This method cooks greens on a rack or in a metal or bamboo steamer basket over boiling or simmering water in a covered pan. Compared to other cooking methods, steaming does the best job of retaining vitamins, minerals and antioxidants in greens. To maximize nutrient retention, add vegetables to the steamer basket after the water has started steaming, cover the pot and then cook until tender-crisp, not soft.

To steam, wash greens but don't dry them. The water that remains on the greens will be enough to steam the vegetables. Place greens in a heavy pan. Larger, firmer greens (e.g., kale, collard greens, Swiss chard) should have 1/4 to 1/2 inch of water added to the bottom of the pan. (You can also use a steamer basket to steam greens.) Cover and simmer over low heat until greens are wilted. Cooking time will vary from 2 to 15 minutes, depending on the size and toughness of the greens.

Microwaving—This method cooks with high-frequency radio waves that cause food molecules to vibrate, creating friction that heats and cooks the food. Because microwaves travel so fast, foods cook very quickly. To microwave, clean greens but don't dry them. Place wet greens in a microwave-safe dish, add 2 to 4 tablespoons of water and cover. Microwave on medium-high for 2 minutes or until tender.

Cruciferous Vegetables

Bok choy ⟶ broccoflower ⟶ broccoli ⟶ broccoli sprouts ⟶ broccolini ⟶ Brussels sprouts ⟶ cabbage ⟶ cauliflower ⟶ rutabaga ⟶ turnip

Eating cruciferous vegetables on a regular basis has been associated with a lower risk of heart attack, stroke and cancers of the breast, lung, colon, prostate and pancreas. These veggies owe their cancer-fighting potential to phytochemicals called glucosinolates. Once consumed, glucosinolates are converted to active compounds called isothiocyanates and indoles, which have anti-cancer, antioxidant and anti-inflammatory effects in the body. One of the most famous isothiocyanates is sulforaphane, a phytochemical that's plentiful in broccoli and broccoli sprouts.

Cruciferous vegetables do more than add cancer-fighting isothiocyanates to your meals. Many are also exceptional sources of vitamin C and fibre. And cruciferous vegetables also supply vitamin A, folate, calcium and potassium. Here's a nutrient breakdown of many cruciferous vegetables.

Notable Nutrients in Cruciferous Vegetables
Per 1/2 cup (125 mL) serving, cooked (unless otherwise indicated)

	Calories	Vit. A (mcg)	Vit. C (mg)	Folate (mcg)	Calcium (mg)	Potassium (mg)
Bok choy	11	190	23	37	84	333
Broccoli	29	81	54	89	33	241
Brussels sprouts (4 sprouts)	30	33	52	50	30	266
Cabbage, raw	9	3	12	16	17	91
Cauliflower	15	1	29	29	10	93

COOKING CRUCIFEROUS VEGETABLES

Steaming, quick sautéing and stir-frying are the healthiest ways to cook cruciferous vegetables to retain their water-soluble nutrients, including vitamin C, folate and thiamin (vitamin B_1). These methods are gentler on nutrients because vegetables don't come into contact with the cooking water. Glucosinolates in cruciferous vegetables are also water soluble and will leach into cooking water during heating. In fact, if you boil your broccoli or cauliflower you'll lose up to 60 percent of these cancer-fighting compounds! Cooking methods that use the least amount of water are best for retaining glucosinolates.

That said, microwaving—which uses little water—can destroy the phytochemicals in cruciferous vegetables. One study found that microwaving broccoli on high power destroyed 97, 74 and 87 percent of three types of antioxidants. Steaming, on the other hand, resulted in a loss of only 11, 0 and 8 percent of the same antioxidants.[1] The high temperature generated by microwave cooking is thought to inactivate an enzyme in cruciferous vegetables that coverts glucosinolates to their active form, isothiocyanates. This enzyme, called myrosinase, is easily destroyed by heat, so cooking cruciferous vegetables can reduce their cancer-fighting potential.

The bottom line: To maximize the amount of isothiocyanates you get from this family of vegetables, steam, quickly sauté or microwave on medium power until still crunchy. Or better yet, enjoy these veggies raw.

Bright Orange Vegetables

Carrots ⚭ sweet potato ⚭ winter squash (acorn, buttercup, butternut, hubbard, pumpkin, spaghetti)

These vegetables are best known for beta-carotene, the pigment that gives them their bright orange colour and gives us potent health benefits. Beta-carotene is important for two reasons. First, once consumed, the body converts some beta-carotene to retinol, an active form of vitamin A. That's why you may have heard beta-carotene called "provitamin A." As a result, foods rich in beta-carotene supply us with some vitamin A. Too little vitamin A can cause night blindness, dry eyes, dry skin, impaired bone growth and a weak immune system. (Night blindness is a condition in which vision is normal in daylight or other strong light but is very weak or completely lost at night or in dim light.)

Second, beta-carotene is a powerful antioxidant, protecting cells in the body from damage caused by free radicals. Its antioxidant properties may help in preventing certain cancers, most notably lung cancer. A diet packed with beta-carotene is also thought to help protect from heart disease by preventing LDL (bad) cholesterol from sticking to artery walls.

There's no official recommended daily intake for beta-carotene but experts contend that consuming 3 to 6 milligrams of beta-carotene each day will help lower the risk of chronic diseases. That's easy to get by eating orange-coloured vegetables! Consider that a medium-sized baked sweet potato packs close to 17 milligrams of beta-carotene and 1/2 cup of cooked carrots has nearly 5!

Beta-Carotene Content of Bright Orange Vegetables

	Beta-carotene (mg)
Sweet potato, baked, 1 medium	16.8
Carrot juice, 1/2 cup (125 mL)	11
Pumpkin, canned, 1/2 cup (125 mL)	8.5
Pumpkin pie, 1 slice	7.4
Carrots, cooked, 1/2 cup (125 mL)	6.5
Carrots, raw, 1/2 cup (125 mL)	4.6
Winter squash, 1/2 cup (125 mL)	2.9

COOKING BRIGHT ORANGE VEGETABLES

Although these foods deliver significant amounts of beta-carotene, carotenoids are fat soluble, which means that they're best absorbed in the body if they're eaten with a little fat or oil. All it takes is 3 to 5 grams of fat (about a teaspoon) in a meal to ensure that the beta-carotene in your veggies is absorbed.

You may have noticed from the chart above that cooking can improve the availability of beta-carotene in foods. For instance, 1/2 cup of cooked carrots has more beta-carotene than the same serving size of raw carrots. However, overcooking can decrease the availability of beta-carotene by altering its shape. To get the most beta-carotene from your vegetables, it's best to lightly steam or sauté them.

FRUIT

Like vegetables, fruits are an outstanding source of fibre, potassium, vitamin C and folate, vital nutrients for maintaining good health and guarding against disease. And many Canadians who eat too few vegetables also eat too little fruit. Many people just don't think to eat a piece of fruit. It's easier to grab a granola bar or a bagel. And most people prefer to satisfy their sweet tooth with cookies or ice cream instead of naturally sweet fruit.

I recommend that you eat *at least* two fruit servings per day. One fruit serving is 1 medium-sized fruit, 1 cup (250 mL) of chopped fruit or berries or 1/2 cup (125 mL) of 100% fruit juice.

(*The Plant-Based Power Diet* outlines serving sizes for many different types of fruit in Part 2.) On *The Plant-Based Power Diet* you'll be eating plenty of this nutritious food each day.

Quick Tips to Increase Your Fruit Intake

- *Keep fruit at work.* Keep apples, bananas, pears and dried fruit on your desk so you'll have a healthy snack handy when you feel hungry.
- *Keep fruit visible.* Decorate your table, kitchen counter or desk with a bowl of fresh fruit. Keeping fruit visible—and within reach—will encourage healthy snacking.
- *Include fruit at breakfast.* For a nutritious breakfast, purée soy milk with berries, banana and a splash of orange juice. Or top a bowl of breakfast cereal with fresh or dried fruit.
- *Serve fruit for dessert.* If you crave sweets after a meal, reach for fruit instead of a decadent treat. Serve fresh fruit salad, fruit kebabs or fruit crisp, or simply eat a piece of fruit out of your hand.
- *Add fruit to salads.* Who says salads have to contain vegetables only? Dried fruit, berries, orange segments, apple slices and pineapple chunks add flavour and a boost of nutrients to green salads.
- *Bake with fruit.* Add fruit to pancakes, waffles, muffins, cookies and pies to increase nutrient and fibre content.
- *Make fruit appealing.* Your family may like fruit better if it's served with a tasty dip like Lemon Maple Glaze (page 216) or low-fat chocolate or vanilla pudding made from soy milk.
- *Garnish with fruit.* Sneak fruit into your family's diet by decorating plates or serving dishes with fruit slices or berries.
- *Consider convenience.* Buy packages of frozen berries or cut up fruit to add to smoothies. Pick up a fresh fruit salad or precut fresh fruit from the deli section of your grocery store.

There's good reason to eat more fruit. A diet rich in colourful, nutrient-dense fruit has been linked to lower rates of cancer, heart disease, stroke, cataract, macular degeneration and type 2 diabetes.

Boosting your intake of fruit can also help control blood pressure and cholesterol, decrease bone loss, promote weight loss and prevent a painful intestinal condition called diverticulitis.

There's no need to limit eating fruit for fear of its sugar content. It's true that fruit contains sugars, mainly fructose, which provides a source of energy. But unlike refined sugars found in candy, baked goods and soft drinks, the sugar in fruit is naturally occurring. These are considered healthy sugars because, along with them, you also get vitamins, minerals, phytochemicals and fibre.

Here are a few superstars that should be included often in *The Plant-Based Power Diet*.

Berries

Açai berries ⚬ blackberries ⚬ blueberries ⚬ cranberries
strawberries ⚬ raspberries

Berries' reputation as "super fruits" comes from their strikingly high antioxidant content. In fact, when researchers measured the antioxidant content of more than 1000 commonly eaten foods, blackberries, strawberries, cranberries, raspberries, blueberries, cranberry juice and blueberry juice were among the top 50 foods containing the most antioxidants per serving.[2]

A handful of phytochemicals contribute to berries' healthy effects. Ellagic acid, plentiful in strawberries and raspberries, acts as an antioxidant, helps the body to deactivate specific carcinogens and slows the growth of cancer cells. *Anthocyanins* give berries their deep red-blue colour. They're abundant in blueberries and cranberries and have been shown in laboratory studies to inhibit the growth of cancer cells. Other phytochemicals in berries called flavonoids and phenolic acids are also believed to have anti-cancer properties.

Flavonoids in berries may also keep your mind sharp as you age. A berry-rich diet can activate the brain's natural housecleaning process, helping to remove toxins and other compounds that can interfere with brain function.

Buying, Storing and Preparing Berries

Fresh berries are very perishable, so purchase them as close to when you intend to use them as possible—up to a few days in advance. Choose berries that are firm, plump and free of mould and that have a uniform colour and a good aroma. Avoid overly soft and dull-coloured berries. (The deeper the colour, the higher the concentration of beneficial anthocyanins.) Make sure there are no signs of moisture, which causes berries to decay.

If you're buying berries packaged in a container, make sure they're not packed too tightly, as this can crush and damage them. When buying frozen berries, shake the bag gently to ensure that the berries move freely. If the berries are clumped together, this may mean they've been thawed and refrozen.

Before storing berries in the refrigerator, remove any damaged or mouldy berries so they won't contaminate others. Store unwashed berries in their original container, covered with plastic wrap. You can also store raspberries and strawberries spread out on a plate covered with a paper towel, and then covered with plastic wrap.

Properly stored in the refrigerator, blueberries will keep for up to one week, although they will be freshest if used within the first few days. Strawberries and raspberries will last for two days. Fresh cranberries can be stored in the fridge for several months. Frozen berries will keep for one year; frozen cranberries can last for several years.

Just before using, place berries in a strainer and briefly rinse under cool running water. That's it—the berries are now ready to enjoy or add to a recipe.

To freeze berries, rinse in a strainer, drain and remove any damaged berries. To ensure uniform texture when they're thawed, spread out the berries on a cookie sheet and place in the freezer until frozen. Then put the berries in a sealable plastic freezer bag and store in the freezer. Don't forget to date the packages.

Citrus Fruit

Grapefruit ✑ lemons ✑ limes ✑ oranges ✑ pomelos ✑ tangerines

A diet high in citrus fruit has been shown to guard against certain cancers and heart disease. And there's more. Citrus fruit may also help lower the risk of arthritis, asthma, macular degeneration, cataracts and cognitive impairment. This category of fruit has plenty to offer on the nutrition front. Citrus fruit, especially oranges, are renowned for vitamin C, a nutrient that bolsters the immune system, fights free radicals and maintains the integrity of body tissues. In fact, one large orange supplies 98 milligrams of vitamin C, more than a full day's requirement!

Citrus fruit have plenty of other protective compounds hiding beneath their fragrant peel. They contain generous amounts of folate, potassium and thiamin as well as some vitamin A, calcium, magnesium and fibre. Pink and red grapefruit also contain lycopene, a phytochemical shown to guard against prostate cancer. Thanks to their flavonoid content, citrus fruit may also help prevent stroke. Flavonoids in oranges and grapefruit have been shown to protect brain cells, strengthen and tone blood vessels and reduce inflammation.

Varieties of Citrus Fruit

Fresh citrus fruit from California, Florida and Arizona is available in Canada throughout the year. Here's a guide to the many varieties of citrus fruit available at produce markets and grocery stores.

- *Navel oranges* are easy to identify; they're the ones with the button formation opposite their stem end. Navel oranges are seedless and have a thick skin, and their flesh is juicy and sweet. Navel oranges are great for making juice, for fruit salads and for snacking (they peel and segment easily).
- *Valencia oranges* are small to medium-sized and may have a few seeds. They're usually thin-skinned and hard to peel. But once peeled, Valencia oranges have a flesh that is juicy and sweet. This orange is well suited for juicing because its flesh contains a great

Notable Nutrients in Citrus Fruit

	Calories	Fibre (g)	Vit. C (mg)	Folate (mcg)	Potassium (mg)
Orange, 1 medium	62	3.1	70	39	237
Orange juice, raw, 1/2 cup (125 mL)	56	0	62	37	248
Grapefruit, pink or red, 1/2	37	1.4	45	11	156
Grapefruit, white, 1/2	39	1.3	39	12	175
Grapefruit juice, raw, 1/2 cup (125 mL)	48	0	47	12	200
Tangerine, 1 medium	47	1.6	23.5	14	146

amount of juice and its thin skin makes it easy to hand squeeze. It's also a good eating orange, containing few or no seeds.

- **Blood oranges** have a bright red to deep maroon interior colour (thanks to their anthocyanins) and an orange-red skin. Their distinctive, strong citrus flavour is sweeter and less acidic than other varieties of oranges. Blood oranges can be used like any other orange but are best used when colour is important. They tend to be small in size, are fairly easy to peel, and have few if any seeds.
- **Seville oranges** have a flattened appearance and a rough, thick skin. The flesh contains a lot of seeds. Seville oranges are bitter tasting and generally not eaten out-of-hand; they are more often used for cooking because of their strong orange flavour. They're popular for making marmalades, jellies and jams and well suited for marinades. They are mostly grown in the Mediterranean regions and have a short growing season, so they are not always readily available.
- **Minneola tangelos** are easily spotted by the knob-like formation at their stem end. This fruit has a deep red-orange skin and a sweet-tart flavour. Minneolas peel very easily and have few if any seeds.

- *Mandarin oranges* are loose skinned and easy to peel. A mandarin's size, shape, colour and flavour will vary with the variety. In general, mandarins are sweet tasting and juicy.
- *Tangerines* are sometimes mistakenly referred to as mandarins but tangerines are actually a subgroup of mandarins. The tangerine is a cross between a mandarin and the bitter orange. There are many different varieties of tangerines; most are smaller in size than an orange and have a slightly flattened shape. Their skins are generally deep reddish-orange, slightly textured, loose fitting and easy to peel. They contain 8 to 15 segments, which are easily separated.
- *Pomelos*, sometimes referred to as Chinese grapefruit, are the largest citrus fruit. They grow to be as big as or bigger than a grapefruit and have a thick green to yellow skin and firm flesh. Interior colour varies from white to deep pink. Pomelos commonly have from 16 to 18 firm, juicy segments, whereas most grapefruit have 12 segments. The taste of pomelo is sweeter and less acidic than grapefruit.
- *Meyer lemons* are favourites of chefs and food lovers, as they are sweeter than regular lemons (e.g., Eureka and Lisbon). When a Meyer lemon's flesh or juice is added to a dish, it adds a sweet and only slightly tart flavor. It has a soft skin that develops an orange hue when the fruit is fully ripe. Its distinctive flavour hints of tangerine; indeed, the Meyer lemon is actually a cross between a lemon and another citrus fruit, possibly an orange or a mandarin. It was introduced to North America from China in 1908 by Frank N. Meyer, a U.S. government employee. Since they require more care when shipping and storing, they are not widely grown on a commercial basis but are occasionally available in specialty food stores.

LEGUMES AND SOY

The nutritional content of legumes—lentils, split peas, chickpeas, kidney beans, black beans, pinto beans, soybeans—is hard to ignore. They're an excellent source of slow-burning carbohydrate and vegetarian protein and they're one of the highest-fibre foods you can eat. For instance, 1 cup of lentils delivers 18 grams of protein (the protein equivalent of three eggs or 2.5 ounces of meat!) and 15 grams of fibre (slightly more than 1/2 cup of bran cereal!).

Legumes are also an excellent source of folate, a B vitamin linked to a healthy pregnancy and a lower risk of colon cancer. Lentils and beans offer calcium, magnesium and potassium, minerals that help keep blood pressure in check. And they're a great source of iron in a plant-based diet. Studies suggest that eating legumes at least four times per week helps lower the risk of heart disease, type 2 diabetes and prostate cancer. Here's how beans and lentils stack up on the nutrition front—very impressively, I might add!

Notable Nutrients in Legumes
Per 3/4 cup (175 mL) serving, cooked

	Calories	Protein (g)	Fibre (g)
Black beans	170	11.4	11.2
Garbanzo beans	202	11	9.3
Kidney beans	169	11.5	8.5
Lentils	172	13.4	11.7
Lima beans	162	11	10
Navy beans	191	11.2	14.3
Pinto beans	183	11.6	11.5
Soybeans	223	21.5	7.7
Edamame	142	12.6	6

	Folate (mcg)	Calcium (mg)	Magnesium (mg)	Iron (mg)
Black beans	192	35	90	2.7
Garbanzo beans	212	60	59	3.6
Kidney beans	173	46	56	3
Lentils	269	28	53	5
Lima beans	117	24	61	3.4
Navy beans	191	94	72	3.2
Pinto beans	221	59	64	2.7
Soybeans	70	132	111	6.6
Edamame	362	73	74	2.6

COOKING WITH BEANS AND LENTILS

Beans and lentils are sold dried and canned. Canned beans and lentils are incredibly convenient because they're already cooked and ready to add to salads, soups, stews, pasta sauces and whole-grain pilafs. But you must drain and rinse canned beans first to remove excess sodium and gas-producing carbohydrates. If you prefer to buy dried beans, they need to be rehydrated and then cooked before eating or adding to recipes.

Soy foods are a special category of legumes that also supply a hefty amount of protein to *The Plant-Based Power Diet*. Soybeans, edamame (young green soybeans in pods), tofu, tempeh, soy "meats" and soy beverages are all included in this food group. Besides protein, vitamins and minerals, soy foods deliver many phytochemicals that protect from disease. The most studied phytochemicals

---

Quick soak and cook instructions for dried beans

Quick soak: Place beans in a large pot with three times the volume of cool water. Bring beans and water to a boil for 2 minutes and then remove from the heat. Cover and let stand for 1 hour. After they have soaked for 1 hour, drain and rinse in a colander.

Cook: Add 3 cups of unsalted water for every 1 cup of soaked beans. The water should be 2 inches (5 cm) above the top of the beans. Add 1 to 2 tablespoons of vegetable oil to prevent boiling over. Bring the beans to a gentle boil and then reduce to a simmer, partially covering the pot. Gently stir beans occasionally during cooking. Skim off any foam that develops during cooking.

Cooking time will vary depending on the size of the legume. Small legumes (black beans, pinto beans, navy beans, lentils) may take 30 to 45 minutes to cook; medium-sized legumes (kidney beans, chickpeas, lima beans) can take 1 to 2 hours.

Once beans are tender, remove from the heat and allow them to sit in cooking liquid while they cool. This prevents them from drying out. Once cooked, legumes are ready to be used in recipes.

in soybeans are called isoflavones. Research strongly suggests that a regular intake of soy isoflavones can help lower the risk of breast cancer, breast cancer recurrence and prostate cancer.

Is Soy Safe to Eat?

As nutritious as soybeans are, you may have read that eating soy is not good for you. Perhaps you've been told that soy increases breast cancer risk or that it disrupts thyroid function. So what's the real deal? Is it safe to include soy foods in a plant-based diet? Yes! And here's why.

The case against soy revolves around isoflavones. The most controversial issue is breast cancer. The concern is that soy isoflavones could increase a woman's total estrogen level and encourage the growth of estrogen-dependent breast cancer, especially in breast cancer survivors. Yet studies suggest that consuming soy reduces breast cancer risk in Asian populations. In Western women, soy hasn't been shown to increase or decrease risk, but that's likely because in North America we don't consume enough soy isoflavones to lower breast cancer risk.

What is becoming clear, however, is that soy may protect breast cancer survivors from having their cancer return. Recent studies have linked soy to improved breast cancer survival in Asian and North American women. A regular soy intake has been found to lower the risk of breast cancer recurrence in women with early and late-stage breast cancer, women with hormone-positive and hormone-negative breast cancer and tamoxifen users and non-users. (Tamoxifen is a drug used to treat hormone-positive early breast cancer.)

Soy foods may protect from breast cancer in a number of ways. Isoflavones may decrease circulating estrogen levels and increase its removal from the body. Soy also contains folate, calcium, fibre, protein and many phytochemicals that individually, or together, may help combat cancer.

What about thyroid health? Toxicologists caution that eating large amounts of soy can result in an underactive thyroid and goiter (an enlarged thyroid gland) by blocking the production of thyroid hormones. However, this appears to occur only in people who

Ways to add soy to *The Plant-Based Power Diet*

Soybeans. Buy them canned or dried; add cooked soybeans to salads, soups, casseroles, chilis and curries.

Edamame. These green young soybeans, still in the pod, can be found in the frozen food aisle of most grocery stores. Boil or steam edamame; add hulled beans to salads and rice dishes or enjoy them hot or cold as a snack.

Soy nuts. They're made from whole soybeans that have been soaked in water and then roasted until crisp and brown. If you have high blood pressure, look for unsalted soy nuts.

Soy flour. Soybeans that are de-fatted and finely ground become soy flour. Replace up to 1/2 cup of all-purpose wheat flour with soy flour in baked-good recipes.

Soy beverages. Unflavoured products contain much less added sugar and more protein than flavoured; unsweetened brands have no added sugar. Use on cereal, in smoothies, in coffee, in soups and in cooking and baking.

Tempeh. These tasty cakes of fermented soybeans are often made with grain and seasoning. Tempeh can be sliced or crumbled and added to stir-fries, casseroles and chilis.

Tofu. Made from soybeans, water and a curdling agent, tofu's mild flavour takes on flavours from spices and marinades. Silken tofu has a soft consistency and is best suited for salad dressings, sauces and desserts. Regular tofu is available soft, medium or firm. Use firm or extra-firm tofu in stir-fries or any dish where you want the tofu to retain its shape.

are deficient in iodine, a mineral that's needed for normal thyroid function. In developed countries, salt is fortified with iodine to prevent deficiency. It's possible, however, that people who eat soy foods and who don't get enough iodine from their diet could be at risk for goiter.

North Americans get enough iodine by using iodized salt and eating fish and dairy products. But because the iodine content of soil varies widely, plant foods aren't always a good source of the mineral. If you don't use iodized salt—and you may not if you're watching your blood pressure—I recommend that you add an iodine supplement to your plant-based diet. All you need is 75 to 150 micrograms four times a week. (Check your multivitamin first to see if it contains iodine.) More isn't necessarily better, since too much iodine can cause thyroid problems as well.

Unless you're allergic to soy, soy foods can be safely consumed as part of a healthy, plant-based diet.

Legumes and soybeans are some of the most versatile, nutritious and inexpensive foods around, yet many people don't eat them on a regular basis. My private-practice clients frequently tell me they don't eat beans often because they don't know what to do with them—aside from making a pot of chili or opening a can of beans in tomato sauce. And many people have never cooked with tofu. *The Plant-Based Power Diet* includes many delicious legume and soy recipes that I guarantee you'll want to make over and over again.

GRAINS

Grain foods like rice, quinoa, millet, oats, corn, pasta and bread add carbohydrate and fibre to a plant-based diet. And if you choose their whole-grain version, they offer a unique package of nutrients and phytochemicals that have multiple health benefits. A wealth of consistent scientific evidence shows that men and women who choose whole grains over their refined cousins have a lower risk of heart disease, stroke and type 2 diabetes.

All grain—be it wheat, rye, oats or spelt—starts out as whole-grain kernels composed of three layers: the outer bran layer where nearly all of the fibre is; the inner germ layer that's rich in nutrients, antioxidants and healthy fats; and the endosperm that contains most of the starch. Eating foods made from whole grains means that you're getting *all* parts of the grain kernel and all of the nutrients, phytochemicals and fibre they contain. In fact, the fibre content of whole grains can be four times that of refined grains!

Key Nutrients and Phytochemicals in Whole Grains

Nutrient	What It Does	Good Sources
Insoluble fibre	Adds bulk to stool and helps prevent constipation, hemorrhoids and diverticulosis and possibly colon cancer.	Whole wheat Brown rice
Soluble fibre	Lowers cholesterol and helps reduce the risk of heart disease and stroke. Helps stabilize blood sugar by slowing the absorption of glucose from the gut. Increases the feeling of fullness after eating and may help prevent weight gain.	Oats, oat bran Barley Rye
Resistant starch	A fibre that encourages the growth of beneficial bacteria to help keep the bowel healthy.	All
Folate	Helps produce and maintain new cells, is needed to make DNA and helps prevent changes to DNA that may lead to cancer.	Fortified whole-grain ready-to-eat cereals
Vitamin E	Antioxidant. Protects cells against harmful effects of free radicals, enhances immune function and helps repair DNA.	All
Magnesium	Helps regulate blood sugar, promotes normal blood pressure and is involved in energy metabolism and bone health.	100% bran Oat bran Brown rice
Selenium	Used to make enzymes in the body that act as antioxidants, enhance immune function and help regulate thyroid function.	Brown rice Whole wheat
Lignans	Lower LDL cholesterol levels and may help prevent heart disease. May reduce risk of breast, ovarian, endometrial and prostate cancers.	Flaxseed
Phytosterols	Lower LDL cholesterol levels and may help prevent coronary heart disease.	Whole wheat

When whole grains are refined, milled, scraped and processed into flakes, puffs or white flour, the bran and germ are removed and all that's left is the starchy endosperm. Without bran and germ, 25 percent of a grain's protein is lost along with at least 17 nutrients. Highly processed grains also contain less fibre and 75 percent fewer phytochemicals. While refined grains are enriched with some—but not all—vitamins and minerals lost through processing, disease-fighting phytochemicals are not added back. What's more, most refined grains have a high glycemic index, meaning that they cause your blood sugar and insulin to spike rapidly. A high glycemic diet can increase the risk of type 2 diabetes as well as breast and colon cancers.

Whole grains are particularly good sources of fibre, folate, vitamin E, magnesium and selenium. The main phytochemicals found in whole grains include compounds called lignans and phyto-sterols. The chart on page 46 outlines important disease-fighting compounds found in whole grains and what they do in the body.

Whole Grains on *The Plant-Based Power Diet*

A whole foods, plant-based diet should include mainly whole grains, rather than refined grains. That doesn't mean you can't eat any refined grains at all; just make sure they make up the minority, not the majority, of grains in your diet. (Here's some good news: Even though they're refined grains, white semolina pasta and white basmati rice have a low glycemic index!) The following is an intro-duction to the world of whole grains. As you'll see, it stretches far beyond brown rice and quinoa!

Amaranth This gluten-free grain originates in South America, where it's a staple foodstuff. Amaranth is gaining popularity in North America for its versatility and unusually high protein content. It's also a good source of dietary fibre, iron, calcium, magnesium, copper and manganese. Amaranth can be cooked as a cereal, popped like popcorn, sprouted or toasted. It's very high in protein and contains high levels of calcium and iron when compared to other cereal grains. Amaranth seeds can also be ground into flour and used in baked goods and pasta.

Barley *(hulled or dehulled)* Barley is reportedly the oldest cultivated cereal and is even thought to predate the cultivation of rice in the Far East. Barley is a versatile grain with a rich nutty flavour and chewy, pasta-like texture. It's an excellent source of fibre and selenium and a good source of phosphorus, copper and manganese. Hulled barley (sometimes called dehulled barley) is the whole-grain version; only the outermost hull of the grain is removed, preserving its nutrient content. Because it's been processed to a lesser degree than pearled barley or pot barley, hulled barley is chewier and requires more soaking and cooking.

Brown rice A staple food for two-thirds of the world's population, rice is a wholesome and nutritious cereal grain that can be made into myriad sweet and savoury dishes. Brown rice, with only the outer layer removed, is a good source of many vitamins and minerals, including fibre, niacin, vitamin B_6, magnesium, manganese, phosphorus and selenium.

Buckwheat A staple in many parts of Europe, this whole grain is eaten widely in the form of kasha, whole groats and soba noodles. Buckwheat is actually not a grain seed. Rather, it's the seed of a fruit that is related to rhubarb and sorrel. That's why buckwheat is a great substitute for people with wheat allergy or gluten intolerance. (It's considered a grain because that's how it is classified in the culinary world.) Buckwheat is sold either unroasted or roasted (kasha). Unroasted buckwheat has a soft, subtle flavour, while roasted buckwheat has an earthy, nutty taste. You can also buy buckwheat ground into flour for baking.

Emmer *(farro)* This ancient strain of wheat was one of the first grains ever domesticated in the Fertile Crescent of the Middle East. It eventually made its way to Italy to become the standard daily ration of the Roman legions. Over the centuries, emmer was gradually abandoned in favour of durum wheat. Today, however, emmer is making a comeback. Also known as farro, the ancient grain is becoming popular with chefs and foodies. Look for farro in specialty food stores. Be sure to buy the whole-grain version: Avoid labels that say "pearled"; look for the words *whole farro*. Use cooked farro in soups, pilafs and whole-grain salads.

Flaxseed Flax is a blue-flowering crop grown on the Canadian prairies for its oil-rich seeds that are tiny, smooth and flat and range in colour from golden to reddish-brown. Flaxseeds are a good source of soluble fibre and alpha-linolenic acid (ALA), an omega-3 fatty acid linked to heart health. Flaxseeds also contain phytochemicals called lignans, compounds thought to help guard against breast cancer.

Grind flaxseeds in a coffee grinder before eating or using in cooking. Otherwise, whole flaxseed may pass through your intestine undigested, which means you won't reap its health benefits. You can purchase flaxseed in bulk—whole or ground—at many grocery stores and health food stores. Ground flaxseeds can be stored in an airtight container for several months and can be added to many foods and recipes.

Kamut Kamut is an ancient relative of modern wheat—durum wheat, to be exact. In fact, *kamut* is an ancient word for wheat. Modern wheat has been altered over the years through breeding to increase its yield and raise its gluten content for commercial baking. Such alterations have made modern wheat more difficult to digest. Because kamut has not been in our food supply long, it has retained many of its original traits and may be easier to digest by some people (but it is not gluten-free). Compared to common wheat, kamut wheat is higher in protein, vitamin E, magnesium, selenium and zinc. Cooked kamut berries have a buttery flavour. You can also find kamut flour and breakfast cereals made with kamut.

Millet (*hulled*) This grain has a long history of cultivation, as it was an important food in Europe in the Middle Ages. Today, millet continues to be a staple in the diet of many African and Asian countries. This tasty, fluffy grain is rich in B vitamins, iron and copper. The tiny, pale yellow or reddish-orange beads can be cooked like any other grain and served with many types of food. The most common type you'll find in stores is hulled millet. Occasionally, you may find cracked millet sold as couscous, although most often couscous is made from semolina, the same type of wheat used to make pasta. Millet is also available as flour in natural food stores.

Oats Oats are an excellent source of soluble fibre, the type that lowers elevated blood cholesterol and helps stabilize blood sugar. In addition, oats are a good source of vitamin B_1 (thiamin), vitamin B_2 (riboflavin) and vitamin E. Oats are available in a variety of forms—from instant to old fashioned to steel cut—lending to their versatility. Oats can be cooked and enjoyed as porridge or incorporated into many recipes. All oats start out as oat groats, the whole grain of the oat, with only the outer hard husk removed. The degree to which oats have been processed determines how long they need to be cooked.

- *Steel-cut oats* are whole oat groats that have been chopped into two or three pieces. Also known as Scotch oats or Irish porridge, steel-cut oats require longer cooking than other oats and remain very chewy (which many people like!).
- *Rolled oats* (old-fashioned oats) are oat groats that have been steamed, rolled and flaked for easier cooking.
- *Quick-cooking oats* are rolled oats that have been chopped into small flakes and take only 3 to 4 minutes to cook.
- *Instant oats* are basically powdered oats. Instant oats cannot be used for cooking or baking. Although they're convenient, most packages of instant oats have added salt and sugar. Choose an instant oatmeal that's low in sugar (ideally unflavoured or no added sugar) and low in salt. Choose brands that contain less than 6 grams of sugar and no more than 250 milligrams of sodium per serving.
- *Oat bran* is not truly a whole grain, but you can consider it as a whole grain since it's a concentrated source of bran that's missing

from refined grains. Oat bran is the outer layer of the oat grain, so it's very high in soluble fibre. It can be cooked to make a nutritious hot breakfast cereal.

- *Oat flour* is available at specialty and health food stores. It's made from oat groats and can be used in baking.

Quinoa Cultivated in the mountain regions of Peru and Chile for more than 5000 years, quinoa was a staple in the native Indian diet. Most commonly considered a grain, quinoa is actually a relative of leafy green vegetables (spinach and Swiss chard). Quinoa is rich in protein and also a good source of calcium and iron. It's fluffy and slightly crunchy and has a somewhat nutty flavour when cooked. It can be eaten plain as a side dish or used as a substitute for rice in casseroles, stuffed peppers, soups, salads and stews. Quinoa can also be eaten as a hot breakfast cereal.

Rye The fact that this grain is hardy enough to grow in very cold climates has made it a staple of Northern Europeans, who use it to make breads, crackers and even whisky. Rye is a high-protein, high-fibre grain of at least equal nutritional quality to wheat flour. It has a distinctive, rich, hearty flavour. Soaked and cooked rye berries are sometimes added to breads for extra texture or used to make pilafs or hot breakfast cereals. Rye flakes are often combined with other grains and then cooked to make a hot breakfast cereal.

Spelt This distant cousin to modern wheat was originally grown in Iran around 5000 to 6000 BC. Spelt has been grown in North America for just over 100 years and is gaining popularity due to its nutty flavour and high nutrient content. Spelt contains more protein than wheat, and the protein in spelt is easier to digest. This means that some people who are allergic to wheat may be able to tolerate spelt. However, spelt contains gluten so it is not suitable for a gluten-free diet.

Spelt berries can be cooked and served as a whole-grain side dish or hot cereal. Spelt flour is available for baking; it has a somewhat nuttier and slightly sweeter flavour than regular whole wheat flour. You can also find spelt products such as bread and pasta in most natural food stores. Be sure to choose products that are made with "whole" spelt.

Teff This whole grain, a type of millet, is a staple food for more than two-thirds of Ethiopians, who make it into a spongy sourdough flatbread. Teff gets its name from its tiny grain size; "teff" comes from *teffa*, meaning "lost" in Amharic. This grain is very high in what's called resistant starch, a type of fibre that helps control blood sugar, manage weight and maintain the health of your colon.

Teff has a sweet, molasses-like flavour and is incredibly versatile. It can be cooked as porridge, used as an ingredient in pancakes, muffins and other baked goods or made into "teff polenta." Teff grains can be red, brown or white. Teff is also making its way into a number of gluten-free products.

Whole wheat In its unrefined state, wheat is a good source of fibre and many vitamins and minerals. Whole wheat comes in many forms other than a loaf of bread. *Wheat berries* are wheat kernels that have been stripped only of their inedible outer hulls. They're a nutritious whole-grain side dish, but they take a long time to cook. Hard wheat berries can be cooked as a cereal, sprouted for salads or milled into flour if you have a home grinder.

If you don't have time to prepare the whole berries, cracked wheat, bulgur or wheat flakes are more convenient alternatives. *Cracked wheat*, as the name implies, is cracked whole wheat kernels. It cooks faster than wheat berries, but not as fast as bulgur. *Bulgur* is made from whole wheat that's been soaked and baked to speed up the cooking time. It's especially popular in the Middle East, where it's used to make tabbouleh and pilafs. Bulgur comes either whole or cracked into fine, medium or coarse grains.

Wild rice This grain isn't actually related to rice at all but is instead the seed of an aquatic grass. It's similar to rice in that both grow in water and produce a grain. Wild rice is the only cereal grain that's native to North America. In its finished form wild rice is a long, slender, coffee-coloured kernel that butterflies open during cooking to reveal a cream-coloured interior. It has a woodsy flavour and chewy texture. Compared to brown rice, wild rice is higher in protein, iron, potassium and zinc. Wild rice can be eaten on its own or used in combination with other rices.

Other Whole-Grain Products

Whole grains are available in many forms: as flours, in cereals, in breads and in crackers. When buying whole grains that have been processed to make another product, be sure to choose the whole-grain version. Look for claims like "100% whole grain." Foods that state "whole grains" on their package may contain only a tiny amount of whole grain. Check the ingredient list, too. Look for a whole grain to be listed first. This means that the product is predominately whole grain. If a whole grain is listed second, you may be getting only a little or nearly half whole grain. Ideally, choose products that are made entirely of whole grains.

LABEL READING 101
Words that always mean whole grain
(these ingredients contain all parts of the grain)
whole-grain whole wheat
whole [name of grain]
stoneground whole [name of grain]
brown rice
oats, oatmeal
wheat berries

Words that may not mean whole grain
(these ingredients may be missing part of the grain)
whole wheat
semolina
durum wheat
organic flour
multigrain

Words that mean refined grain
(these ingredients may be missing part of the grain)
wheat flour
unbleached wheat flour
cornmeal
wheat germ

SPROUTED GRAINS

You may have noticed breads made from sprouted grains in the grocery store. These products are made from whole grains that have been exposed to just the right temperature and amount of moisture so the germ inside the grain sprouts. These sprouted grains are then used to bake bread. Proponents of sprouted whole grains claim they're more nutritious than regular whole grains. They're said to have more fibre, protein, vitamin C and B vitamins. They also contain natural enzymes, which can improve digestion. And sprouted grain breads may also contain less gluten, the protein that lends structure to bread. You don't have to rely on retail products to add sprouted grains to your diet. Look for sprouted grain flours to use in baking in natural and specialty food stores.

COOKING WITH WHOLE GRAINS

On *The Plant-Based Power Diet* I encourage you to enjoy a variety of whole grains served on their own, as hot cereals, as pilafs and in stir-fries and casseroles. Many of my clients complain that they don't have time on a busy weekday morning to cook a pot of steel-cut oats for breakfast. Or that spending 45 minutes or more to cook brown rice or wheat berries isn't conducive to getting dinner on the table in a hurry. One solution: Cook a batch of whole grains on the weekend when you have more time. Refrigerate and then reheat in the microwave or steamer to enjoy over the next few days. Or freeze in small portions to use in other recipes.

It's important to thoroughly rinse all grains under running water before cooking to remove any dirt or debris. (You don't have to rinse oats.) Kamut berries, spelt berries, rye berries and wheat berries must be soaked before cooking. Soaking softens the grain kernel so cooking time is reduced. To soak, place rinsed berries in a bowl and cover with 2 inches (5 cm) of water. Let soak for 8 hours or overnight. Once soaked, berries are ready to cook according to the instructions in the table below.

Use water or low-sodium vegetable broth for cooking liquid. To add flavour to cooked grains, add a bay leaf to simmering grains.

A Quick Guide to Cooking Whole Grains

Type of Grain	Grain-to-Liquid Ratio	Cooking Time (approx.)
Amaranth	1 part rice to 3 parts liquid. Combine amaranth and water in saucepan. Bring to boil. Cover, reduce heat and let simmer until cooked. 1 cup dry yields 2 1/2 cups cooked.	20 to 25 minutes
Barley (hulled)	1 part barley to 3 1/2 parts liquid. Add barley and liquid to saucepan. Bring to boil, reduce heat, cover and simmer until cooked. 1 cup dry yields 3 cups cooked.	60 to 90 minutes
Brown rice (long grain)	1 part rice to 2 parts liquid. Bring rice and liquid to a boil in a saucepan. Reduce heat, cover and simmer until cooked. To cook brown basmati rice, soak it in a bowl of cool water before cooking, stirring frequently and replacing the water four times or until the water no longer has a milky appearance. 1 cup dry yields 3 cups cooked.	40 to 45 minutes
Buckwheat groats (kasha)	1 part buckwheat to 2 parts liquid. Add buckwheat to boiling liquid. Return to a boil, reduce heat, cover and simmer until tender. 1 cup dry yields 3 1/2 cups cooked.	30 minutes

Type of Grain	Grain-to-Liquid Ratio	Cooking Time (approx.)
Bulgur	1 part bulgur to 2 parts liquid. Add bulgur to cold water. Bring to a boil, cover and simmer until tender. 1 cup dry yields 2 1/2 cups cooked.	12 to 15 minutes
Kamut berries	1 part kamut to 3 parts liquid. Add soaked and drained kamut berries to liquid. Cover and simmer until tender but chewy. If grains were not soaked, allow 45 to 60 minutes. 1 cup dry yields 4 cups cooked.	30 to 40 minutes
Millet (hulled)	1 part millet to 2 1/2 parts liquid. Add millet and liquid to saucepan. Bring to boil, reduce heat, cover and simmer until tender and fluffy. 1 cup dry yields 4 cups cooked.	25 minutes
Oats (old fashioned)	1 part oats to 2 parts liquid. Bring water and salt to a boil. Add rolled oats, reduce heat and cook to desired consistency, stirring occasionally. Cover, remove from heat and let stand 5 minutes before serving. 1 cup dry yields 2 cups cooked.	10 to 20 minutes
Oats (steel cut)	1 part oats to 4 parts liquid. Add steel-cut oats to boiling water. When the porridge is smooth and beginning to thicken, reduce heat and simmer, stirring occasionally. 1 cup dry yields 3 cups cooked.	30 minutes
Quinoa	1 part quinoa to 2 parts liquid. Add quinoa and liquid to saucepan. Bring to a boil, reduce heat, cover and simmer until grains are tender and translucent. 1 cup dry yields 3 cups cooked.	15 minutes

Type of Grain	Grain-to-Liquid Ratio	Cooking Time (approx.)
Rye berries	1 part rye to 2 1/2 parts liquid. Add soaked and drained rye berries to boiling water. Reduce heat, cover and simmer until tender. 1 cup dry yields 2 1/2 cups cooked.	60 to 90 minutes
Rye flakes	1 part rye flakes to 2 1/2 parts liquid. Add rye flakes to boiling water. Reduce heat, cover and simmer. 1 cup dry yields 2 1/2 cups cooked.	30 minutes
Spelt berries	1 part spelt to 3 parts liquid. Add soaked and drained spelt berries and liquid to saucepan. Bring to a boil, cover and reduce heat to simmer until tender but chewy.	60 minutes
Wheat berries (hard winter)	1 part wheat berries to 5 parts liquid. Add soaked and drained wheat berries to boiling water and bring to a boil. Reduce heat, cover and simmer. Cook, stirring occasionally until tender but still chewy, adding more water if needed. 1 cup dry yields 2 1/2 cups cooked.	55 to 65 minutes
Wild rice	1 part rice to 3 1/2 parts liquid. Bring rice and liquid to a boil in a saucepan. Cover, reduce heat and cook until the rice grains have "butterflied" (split open and curled). Turn off the heat and let stand covered for 5 minutes. 1 cup dry yields 3 to 4 cups cooked.	40 to 60 minutes

You'll notice that I've included starchy vegetables in this food group. That's because vegetables such as potatoes, yams, winter squash and parsnips contain starch and, as a result, are similar to grains calorically.

HEALTHY FATS AND OILS

Fat that occurs naturally in foods and fat that's added to foods provide essential fatty acids and helps your body absorb fat-soluble vitamins A, D, E and K. Essential fatty acids must be supplied from your diet because your body can't make them on its own. One, called alpha-linolenic acid (ALA), has anti-inflammatory actions in your body and may guard against heart disease. (You'll learn more about these important fats in Step 6.) The following are sources of healthy fats that can be added to a plant-based diet.

Healthy Fats in *The Plant-Based Power Diet*
• Avocado
• Cold pressed oils such as extra virgin olive, flaxseed and canola
• Chia seeds
• Flaxseed
• Hemp seeds
• Nuts and seeds
• Nut and seed butters
• Olives

Added fats and oils are not essential in a plant-based diet. In fact, many experts in plant-based nutrition believe that your fat intake should be kept at a very low level, no more than 10 percent of your daily calories. But small amounts of the right types of fat can fit into *The Plant-Based Power Diet*. Ideally, choose fats in their whole food form—rather than as processed oils—since they also add nutrients and phytochemicals to your diet. Here's how selected fats and oil compare in terms of nutrition.

Nutritional Characteristics of Healthy Fats

Per 1 tablespoon (15 mL), unless otherwise stated.

	Calories	Vitamin E (mg)	Vitamin K (mcg)	ALA (g)
Almond butter	98	3.9	0	0
Avocado, 1/3 whole fruit	107	1.4	14.1	0.08
Canola oil	125	2	17.3	1.32
Chia seeds, whole	35	0.04	0	1.3
Flaxseed oil	122	2	0	7.74
Flaxseed, ground	37	0.2	0.3	1.6
Olive oil	121	2	8.2	0.11
Walnut oil	122	0	2.1	1.43

In Part 2, you'll find *The Plant-Based Power Diet* meal plan. I'll tell you how many servings of each food group you need, what a serving size is, what vitamin supplements to consider and so on. But before you embark on *The Plant-Based Power Diet*, the following chapters are must-reads! They address many of the questions people often ask about a plant-based diet.

Get All of Your Protein from Plant Sources

"If you don't eat meat, where do you get your protein from?" This is likely the first question you'll be asked about your plant-based diet. Perhaps you're wondering the same thing. Many people assume that only animal foods have protein. Or they believe that the protein in plant foods is somehow inferior to animal protein. These are myths! I am happy to tell you that a plant-based diet can easily provide all of the protein your body needs each day!

VITAL PROTEIN

The protein you get from foods—animal and plant—performs many crucial roles in your body. But before it can get to work, food protein is broken down into its individual amino acid building blocks during the process of digestion. These amino acids are then stored in a pool, ready to be repackaged into 10 000 to 50 000 different kinds of body proteins, each one having its own unique role. Protein in the body is used to synthesize and maintain your muscles, connective tissue, skin, tendons, ligaments, bones and teeth. It's also used to make hormones that regulate hundreds of bodily processes. For example, thyroid hormones control your metabolic rate, the speed at which your body burns calories. Hormones called insulin and glucagon closely regulate the level of sugar in your bloodstream.

Enzymes that control billions of chemical reactions taking place in your body every day are also made from protein. And your immune system depends on a constant supply of protein. Amino acids from protein are used to make antibodies, molecules that prevent infection by attacking foreign invaders. Protein also helps maintain fluid balance, transports nutrients in your bloodstream, aids in blood clotting and enables you to transform light into visual images. And if you don't eat enough calories, your body can use protein for energy, too. With all of these important duties, it's no wonder we're so obsessed with getting enough protein in our diet.

How Much Protein Do You Need?

The truth is you don't need as much protein as you may think. You need to consume enough protein each day to make up for the amount your body loses. The amount of protein in your diet has to match the amount you lose in urine, skin, hair and nails and in your muscles during exercise. If you eat more than your daily requirement, excess protein is stored as body fat (not muscle!). Growing children and pregnant and breastfeeding women have higher protein needs because they need to cover daily losses and support growth. Your protein requirements are based on your body weight and expressed in grams of protein per kilogram of body weight.

Our official protein recommendations include a safety factor to cover the needs of most people. However, many experts recommend that people who eat a 100 percent plant-based diet multiply the official Recommended Daily Allowance (RDA) by 10 to 15 percent to account for the different amino acid mixes in plant foods and the fact that some plant proteins are digested less efficiently than animal proteins.

Recommeded Daily Intakes for Protein

	Meat eaters[1]	Plant-based eaters
Adults	0.8 g/kg/day	0.9 g/kg/day
Children, 1 to 3 years	1.0 g/kg/day	1.15 g/kg/day
Children, 4 to 13 years	0.95 g/kg/day	1.1 g/kg/day
Teenagers, 14 to 18 years	0.85 g/kg/day	1.0 g/kg/day
During pregnancy	1.1 g/kg/day	1.25 g/kg/day
While breastfeeding	1.3 g/kg/day	1.5 g/kg/day

Adults who eat a 100 percent plant-based diet require 0.9 grams of protein for every kilogram they weigh. For ease of calculation, it's fine to round up to 1 g/kg/day. (To convert your weight to kilograms, simply divide your weight in pounds by 2.2.) So just how much protein do plant-based eaters need to eat each day? Here are a few examples:

- If you weigh 135 lb (61 kg)
  61 kg × 1 = 61 grams of protein
- If you weigh 150 lb (68 kg)
  68 kg × 1 = 68 grams of protein
- If you weigh 175 lb (79.5 kg)
  79.5 kg × 1 = 79.5 grams of protein
- If you weigh 205 lb (93 kg)
  93 kg × 1 = 93 grams of protein

There's another way to look at how much protein you should be eating each day: as a percentage of your total daily calories. The U.S.-based Institute of Medicine, the organization that sets nutrient RDAs for North Americans, states that it's acceptable for protein to provide anywhere from 10 to 35 percent of your day's worth of calories. This range of protein intake is associated with a lower risk of chronic disease and at the same time provides adequate protein. If you consume below or above this range, there's a potential increase in the risk of chronic diseases and you are also getting too little—or too much—protein. And guess what? Studies show that plant-based eaters typically get 10 to 12 percent of their daily calories from protein.

Protein in a Plant-Based Diet

Nearly all plant foods—grains, vegetables, beans, lentils, nuts and seeds—contain protein. Even many types of fruit have protein, although typically much less than other plant foods. Beans, lentils, soybeans, soy foods, nuts and nut butters are very good sources of protein, rivalling many animal foods. Here's how plant foods stack up when it comes to protein.

Protein Content of Selected Plant Foods

	Protein (g)
Legumes and soy foods	
Baked beans, cooked, 1 cup (250 mL)	14.0
Black beans, cooked, 1 cup (250 mL)	15.2
Kidney beans, cooked, 1 cup (250 mL)	13.3
Lentils, cooked, 1 cup (250 mL)	18.0
Soybeans, cooked, 1 cup (250 mL)	22.2
Soy ground round, cooked, 1/3 cup (75 mL)	10.0
Soy beverage, plain, 1 cup (250 mL)	8.0
Soy nuts, roasted, 1/4 cup (50 mL)	15.0
Tofu, firm, 3/4 cup (175 mL)	15.5
Veggie dog, 1 small (55 g)	8.0
Veggie burger, 1 (75 g)	14.0
Nuts and seeds	
Almonds, 1/4 cup (50 mL)	7.6
Almond butter, 2 tbsp (25 mL)	6.7
Mixed nuts, 1/4 cup (50 mL)	6.0
Peanuts, 1/4 cup (50 mL)	9.4
Peanut butter, 2 tbsp (25 mL)	8.0
Pumpkin seeds, 1/4 cup (50 mL)	8.8
Sunflower seeds, 1/3 cup (75 mL)	6.2
Tahini (sesame butter), 2 tbsp (25 mL)	5.0
Walnuts, 1/4 cup (50 mL)	4.5
Grains	
Amaranth, cooked, 1 cup (250 mL)	9.3
Barley, cooked, 1 cup (250 mL)	3.6
Bran Flakes, 1 cup (250 mL)	3.7
Bread, mixed grain, 2 slices	7.6
Bread, whole wheat pita pocket, 1 large	6.0
Brown rice, cooked, 1 cup (250 mL)	5.0
Buckwheat groats (kasha), cooked, 1 cup (250 mL)	5.7

	Protein (g)
Kamut, cooked, 1 cup (250 mL)	11.0
Millet, cooked, 1 cup (250 mL)	6.1
Oatmeal, cooked, 1 cup (250 mL)	6.0
Quinoa, cooked, 1 cup (250 mL)	8.1
Spaghetti noodles, cooked, 1 cup (250 mL)	8.1
Grain-based beverages	
Almond milk, 1 cup (250 mL)	1.0–2.0
Oat milk, 1 cup (250 mL)	3.0
Rice milk, 1 cup (250 mL)	0.5–2.0
Fruit and vegetables	
Apple, 1 large	0.6
Banana, 1 large	1.5
Blueberries, 1 cup (250 mL)	1.1
Mango, 1	2.7
Asparagus, 8 spears	3.0
Broccoli, cooked, 1 cup (250 mL)	1.9
Carrot sticks, raw, 1 cup (250 mL)	1.1
Potato, Russet, baked, 1	3.0
Red pepper, 1 medium	1.2
Sweet potato, baked, 1 medium	2.3
Vegetable juice, 1 cup (250 mL)	2.0

Source: USDA National Database for Standard Reference, Release 25. USDA Agricultural Research Service. National Agricultural Library. 2012.

Can a Plant-Based Diet Provide Enough Protein?

Yes! Studies conducted on vegetarian populations have shown that protein and calorie intakes are right on target. In fact, the typical protein intake of vegetarians and vegans meets—or exceeds!—daily requirements. Take a look at how easy it is to meet your daily protein requirements with a day's worth of plant-based meals.

Protein in a Plant-Based Menu

	Protein (g)
Breakfast	
Oatmeal, cooked, 1 cup (250 mL)	5.9
Ground flaxseed, 2 tbsp (25 mL)	0.02
Blueberries, 3/4 cup (175 mL)	0.75
Soy beverage, plain, 1 cup (250 mL)	7.0
Tea	0.0
Breakfast total	*13.7*
Snack	
1 apple	0.3
15 almonds	3.2
Snack total	*3.5*
Lunch	
Large green salad with chickpeas	
2 cups (500 mL) mixed greens	0.76
1/2 cup (125 mL) sliced mushrooms	1.08
1/2 cup (125 mL) cherry tomatoes	0.76
1/2 yellow pepper, chopped	0.6
3/4 cup (175 mL) chickpeas	11.0
Whole-grain pumpernickel bread, 1 slice	2.5
Hummus, 2 tbsp (25 mL)	2.2
Water	0.0
Lunch total	*18.9*
Snack	
Soy smoothie	
3/4 cup (175 mL) vanilla soy beverage	5.8
1/2 banana	0.0
1/2 cup (125 mL) frozen raspberries	0.0
Snack total	*5.8*

	Protein (g)
Dinner	
Tofu veggie stir-fry	
Firm tofu, chopped, 3/4 cup (175 mL)	15.5
1 carrot	0.7
1/2 red pepper	0.6
1/2 cup (125 mL) broccoli florets	1.1
1/2 cup (125 mL) snow peas	1.2
Quinoa, cooked, 3/4 cup (175 mL)	6.1
Water	0.0
Dinner total	**25.2**
Total protein intake for the day	**67 grams**

This day's worth of plant-based meals provides 67 grams of protein—enough for a 150 lb (68 kg) adult. Now, what about a 190-pound guy who needs more protein, 86 grams' worth to be precise? (The math: 190 lb [86 kg]: 86 × 1 g/kg = 86 g of protein.) The following easy modifications to the menu above will get him to this daily protein target and increase his calorie intake.

BREAKFAST
• Add 1 slice of whole-grain toast with 1 tablespoon (15 mL) of almond butter for an extra 7.1 grams of protein.

LUNCH
• Increase portion of chickpeas to 1 cup (250 mL) to add 4 grams of protein.

DINNER
• Increase portions of tofu to 1 cup (250 mL) and quinoa to 1 1/2 cups (375 mL) for an additional 11 grams of protein.

These few small adjustments add an extra 22 grams of protein and bring the total daily protein intake to 89 grams! (Keep in mind that more food may need to be added to meet the calorie requirements of our 190-pound male.) Vegan energy bars and vegan protein powders are other ways to bump up your protein intake, although I recommend trying to meet protein needs first by eating whole foods. You'll get more fibre, vitamins, minerals and phytochemicals by doing so. The bottom line: A plant-based diet easily provides enough protein. As long as you eat a variety of foods and include a few plant protein powerhouses—beans, lentils, tofu, veggie burgers, quinoa, etc.—there's no need to worry about protein.

It's also important to meet your daily calorie requirements. If your calorie intake is too low, some of the protein in your diet will be used for energy purposes rather than to make proteins in the body. If you are dieting to lose weight or if your calorie intake is low for another reason, I recommend adding a few extra protein-rich foods to your diet each day.

Do You Need to Combine Proteins?

The notion of protein combining—eating certain plant foods together in the same meal (e.g., grains and beans)—was introduced in the 1970s by Frances Moore Lappé's *Diet for a Small Planet*. The goal was to consume the perfect mix of amino acids at meals, in particular *essential amino acids*. Protein-rich foods supply your body with 20 amino acids, all of which are needed for good health. Your body's actual requirement is for amino acids, not for protein per se. Eleven of these amino acids can be manufactured by your body and are called *non-essential amino acids*. The remaining nine, however, must be supplied by your diet because your body cannot synthesize them on its own. As you may have guessed, they are called *essential amino acids (EAAs)*. If your diet does not supply enough of these essential amino acids, the rate of protein building slows down. Eventually your body breaks down its own proteins (remember those muscle tissues, hormones and enzymes!) to get these amino acids.

Amino Acids in Foods

Essential amino acids (EAAs)	Non-essential amino acids
Histidine	Alanine
Isoleucine	Arginine
Leucine	Asparagine
Lysine	Aspartic acid
Methionine	Cysteine
Phenylalanine	Glutamic acid
Threonine	Glutamine
Tryptophan	Glycine
Valine	Proline
	Serine
	Tyrosine

Animal and plant proteins have different amino acid profiles. Animal protein foods contain all EAAs in sufficient quantities to support growth, repair and maintenance of body tissues. For this reason, animal proteins are considered *complete proteins*. Plant proteins, on the other hand, are low in one or more of the nine EAAs. In some cases, a plant food may even be totally lacking an EAA. The proteins from plant foods are considered *incomplete proteins* for this reason.

So, back to the 1970s. Lappé's book advised strict vegetarians to combine a plant food low in an EAA with another containing a large amount of that EAA. By doing so, vegetarians would be able to consume all nine amino acids that are essential to their bodies. When two or more vegetarian protein foods are combined in this way, they are called *complementary proteins*. For example, legumes, which are low in methionine, could be eaten with nuts or seeds, which are a good source of this amino acid. Legumes could be combined with grains to provide the lysine and threonine missing from beans.

Sounds pretty complicated, right? It was. The good news is that we now know it isn't necessary to combine proteins at meals. As long as you eat a variety of plant foods throughout the day, your body will get all of the amino acids it needs to create those vital body proteins. If you eat only a few foods and your diet lacks variety, you probably won't get enough protein and EAAs. Here's something else to consider: Your body can't tell the difference between EAAs from animal foods and plant foods. They're exactly the same. In fact, plant foods are the original source of all EAAs. Think about it. The EAAs you get from beef and milk ultimately came from the grass or grains that cows grazed on. The same goes for fish that fed on smaller fish that fed on seaweed. The bottom line: Essential amino acids in plant proteins are no different from the EAAs in animal foods.

CAN ATHLETES GET ENOUGH PROTEIN ON A PLANT-BASED DIET?

If you're serious about exercise, you're probably no stranger to protein. Protein-rich foods, protein bars and protein shakes are often recommended by personal trainers to help bulk up and recover from exercise. During the 1800s, it was widely believed that protein was the main fuel burned during exercise. But gone are the days when athletes downed pre-competition meals of eggs and steak. Today we know that almost all of the energy used to fuel exercise—be it weight training, running, tennis or basketball—comes from carbohydrates and fat.

Even so, protein is a very important nutrient in an athlete's diet. Amino acids from protein-rich foods are needed to support muscle rebuilding and repair. Strength athletes break down some muscle tissue during heavy weightlifting. Even endurance athletes such as long distance runners and triathletes burn some protein in their muscles for energy. So it's important for all athletes—vegetarian or not—to get enough protein in their diet to allow muscles to recover after exercise. Adequate protein helps athletes to train hard day after day and stay injury-free.

These extra demands for protein increase an athlete's requirements for the nutrient. To account for the fact that plant proteins are digested less well than animal proteins, athletes who follow a plant-based diet require a little more protein than meat eaters—about

1.3 to 1.8 grams of protein per kilogram of body weight. That means a 175-pound (79.5 kg) marathoner needs roughly 119 grams of protein per day (79.5 kg × 1.5 g/kg/day). Here's how it can be done!

Protein in a Plant-Based Athlete's Menu

	Protein (g)
Breakfast	
Oatmeal, cooked, 2 cups (250 mL)	12.0
Ground flaxseed, 2 tbsp (25 mL)	0.02
Blueberries, 3/4 cup (175 mL)	0.75
Soy beverage, plain, 1 cup (250 mL)	8.0
1 slice toast with 1 tbsp (15 mL) almond butter	7.1
Tea	0.0
Breakfast total	**27.9**
Snack	
1 apple	0.3
15 almonds	3.2
Snack total	**3.5**
Lunch	
Large green salad with chickpeas	
2 cups (500 mL) mixed greens	0.76
1/2 cup (125 mL) sliced mushrooms	1.08
1/2 cup (125 mL) cherry tomatoes	0.76
1/2 yellow pepper, chopped	0.6
1 cup (250 mL) chickpeas	15.0
Whole-grain bagel, 1 medium	11.0
Hummus, 4 tbsp (50 mL)	4.4
Water	0.0
Lunch total	**33.6**

	Protein (g)
Snack	
Soy smoothie	
1 cup (250 mL) vanilla soy beverage	8.0
1 banana	1.5
1/2 cup (125 mL) frozen raspberries	0.75
Snack total	*10.3*
Dinner	
Tofu veggie stir-fry	
Firm tofu, chopped, 1 cup (250 mL)	20.5
1 carrot	0.7
1/2 red pepper	0.6
1/2 cup (125 mL) broccoli florets	1.1
1/2 cup (125 mL) snow peas	1.2
Quinoa, cooked, 2 1/2 cups (625 mL)	20.2
Water	0.0
Dinner total	*44.3*
Total protein intake for the day	*119 grams*

Protein Supplements

As long as athletes eat enough calories and a variety of plant-based protein foods, it's entirely possible to meet protein needs without using protein bars or special supplements. That being said, some athletes will benefit from a plant-based protein powder. It's easy to add to fruit smoothies and soy shakes or mix into a bowl of hot cereal. Vegan Proteins+ by Genuine Health, for example, delivers 20 grams of plant-based protein per scoop. Vega Sport Performance Protein, formulated by professional Ironman triathlete Brendan Brazier, contains 26 grams of plant protein per serving (from yellow pea, brown rice, hemp and alfalfa proteins). Plant-based protein bars are also available and can be used as pre- or post-workout snacks.

Creatine Supplements

There's another supplement that certain athletes may need to consider: creatine supplements. Creatine is made in the body from amino acids and also comes from the diet, mainly from meat and fish. About 95 percent of creatine in your body is stored in your muscles, where it's used to generate energy compounds called ATP (adenosine triphosphate). Exercise that involves brief, intense efforts—weightlifting, sprinting, wrestling—relies heavily on ATP for fuel since it is the only form of energy that muscles can generate at a fast enough rate. But muscles can only provide ATP at maximal rates for a few seconds before their creatine stores become depleted. For this reason, it's thought that athletes who increase their muscle creatine levels by taking creatine supplements will have more energy to perform high-intensity tasks. Since athletes who eat a plant-based diet likely have lower muscle stores of creatine, supplements may be beneficial.

Indeed, studies have shown that creatine supplementation improves performance of brief high-intensity exercise lasting less than 30 seconds. For example, strength athletes who use creatine supplements can complete more repetitions per set of a given exercise and recover more quickly between sets. Creatine supplements don't work for everyone, however. It's thought that some athletes may be more predisposed to store creatine in their muscles than others.

Vitamin B_{12} and Athletes

Another potential issue is vitamin B_{12}, which is found only in animal foods and fortified plant beverages like soy, rice and almond milks. Vitamin B_{12} is important for endurance athletes since it's needed to make red blood cells. (Red blood cells carry oxygen to working muscles.) You'll learn more about vitamin B_{12}—and how to get enough of it in a plant-based diet—in Step 8.

Quick Tips for Meeting Protein Needs

- Be sure to meet your daily calorie requirements. If you are following a low-calorie weight-loss diet or if your calorie intake is low for any other reason, include two additional high-protein foods to your diet.
- Use the chart on page 63 to include a variety of whole plant foods in your daily diet.
- Include legumes and/or soy in at least two meals per day. I'll outline serving sizes in Part 2, *The Plant-Based Power Diet*.
- If you use plant-based beverages, choose soy milk most often. Rice, almond, oat and hemp beverages are low in protein.
- Add whole grains to every meal. Cooked grains such as quinoa, kamut, millet and amaranth are good sources of protein.
- Include nuts and seeds in your diet each day. Eat them as a snack, sprinkle over cereal, add to salads or toss in a stir-fry.
- Use higher-protein spreads such as nut butters, hummus and tahini on bread.
- Consider using a plant-based protein supplement if you feel that your diet does not provide enough protein.

Step 5

Know Your Carbohydrates: Grains, Gluten and More

One thing is certain: Plant-based eaters are not carb phobic! That's because a plant-based diet typically gets 60 percent or more of its calories from carbohydrates. That's a good thing since our bodies need carbohydrates to perform at their peak. Carbohydrates provide about half of all energy that your muscles, nerves and other body tissues use. Your brain relies on a steady supply of carbs to function properly, too. If it weren't for carbohydrates in your diet, you wouldn't have the energy to work out at the gym or to concentrate at the office.

In a plant-based diet, fruit, starchy vegetables, grains, legumes, soy foods and nuts all deliver energy-boosting carbohydrates. These healthy foods supply your body with carbohydrates plus a whole lot more: fibre, vitamins, minerals and hundreds of phytochemicals that fend off disease.

There's a lot of confusion about carbs these days. To many people the word *carbohydrate* means refined starchy foods like white bread, white rice and pasta. As a result, carbohydrate-rich foods are often deemed unhealthy foods that should be avoided. Yet refined starchy foods make up only one category of carbohydrate-rich foods. Other foods that contain carbs are incredibly healthy additions to any diet—plant-based or not.

The term *carbohydrate* encompasses sugars (naturally occurring and refined), starches and fibre. Here's a quick review of carbohydrate basics.

SUGARS: THE GOOD AND THE BAD

Often called simple sugars, these carbohydrates are single sugar molecules (glucose, fructose, galactose) or pairs of two sugar molecules linked together (sucrose, lactose, maltose). Sugars can be naturally occurring (e.g., fructose in fruit, lactose in milk) or added to foods during processing. You'll find naturally occurring sugars in fruit, tomatoes, sweet potatoes, winter squash, carrots, parsnips, peas and turnips. These natural sugars are good for you because they also provide fibre, nutrients and antioxidants.

The sugars you want to limit as much as possible are added sugars. These are refined sugars that go by many different names, including sucrose, glucose, dextrose, liquid sugar, honey, fructose and high-fructose corn syrup. While there's no evidence that sugar causes diabetes, heart disease, cancer or hyperactivity, too much can add a surplus of calories to your diet and promote weight gain. Consuming too much sugar can also raise blood triglycerides, fats that are linked to heart disease. How much sugar is too much? Current recommendations are to limit added sugars to less than 100 calories per day (25 grams or 6 teaspoons' worth) for women and 150 calories (37 grams or 9 teaspoons' worth) for men. (Four grams of sugar is equivalent to 1 teaspoon.)

The most controversial added sugar is high-fructose corn syrup, an inexpensive sweetener that's added to soft drinks, fruit drinks, baked goods and canned fruit. Researchers have linked our increased use of corn syrup sweeteners over the past two decades to rising obesity rates. This correlation doesn't prove that high-fructose corn syrup causes weight gain, but many experts contend that the body metabolizes fructose in high-fructose corn syrup differently than glucose in cane or beet sugar. Fructose doesn't trigger hormone responses that regulate appetite and satiety, which could lead to overeating. Fructose-sweetened beverages have also been shown to impair how the body clears blood sugar and handles fat—detrimental effects that can increase the risk of heart disease and heart attack.

STARCHES: WHOLE VERSUS REFINED

Unlike sugars, starches are complex chains of hundreds or thousands of sugar (glucose) units linked together. You'll find plenty of starch in grains and grain products like breads, cereals, rice, quinoa, millet, pasta and corn. Potatoes and beans and lentils have starch, too.

All grain—be it wheat, rye, oats or spelt—starts out as whole-grain kernels composed of three layers: the outer bran layer where nearly all of the fibre is, the inner germ layer that's rich in nutrients, antioxidants and healthy fats and the endosperm that contains most of the starch. Eating foods made from whole grains means you're getting *all* parts of the grain kernel—and all of the fibre, nutrients and phytochemicals it contains.

When whole grains are refined, milled, scraped and heat processed into flakes, puffs or white flour, the bran and germ are removed and all that's left is the starchy endosperm. Without the bran and germ, about 25 percent of a grain's protein is lost, along with at least 17 nutrients. Refined grains also contain less fibre, vitamins and minerals and 75 percent fewer phytochemicals! Refined flours are enriched with some, but not all, of the vitamins and minerals lost through processing. However, disease-fighting phytochemicals are not added back to refined grains.

As you have probably already guessed, *The Plant-Based Power Diet* is based on whole-grain, not refined, starchy foods! Nutritional benefits aside, eating more whole grains is linked with a lower risk of developing heart disease, type 2 diabetes and breast, colon and prostate cancers. Whole-grain eaters also tend to have healthier body weights than people who eat few whole grains. They also have lower levels of inflammatory chemicals in their bloodstream.

FIBRE: CUTTING THROUGH THE CHAFF

A whole foods, plant-based diet is loaded with dietary fibre. To many people, fibre is synonymous with bran cereal. But if you rely on a single food to get your fibre, you're shortchanging yourself. That's because foods provide two types of fibre: soluble and insoluble.

Both types are present in varying proportions in different foods, but some foods may be rich in one type or the other.

Soluble fibre dissolves in water. It's found in dried peas, beans and lentils, oats, barley, psyllium husks, apples and citrus fruits. When you consume these foods, soluble fibre forms a gel in your stomach and slows the rate of digestion and absorption. Consuming more soluble fibre can help improve blood sugar control and lower LDL (bad) cholesterol.

Foods like wheat bran, whole grains, nuts and vegetables contain mainly *insoluble fibre*. This fibre doesn't dissolve in water, but it does have a significant capacity for retaining water. In this way insoluble fibre increases stool bulk and promotes regularity. By preventing constipation, a high-fibre diet can ease symptoms of irritable bowel syndrome, help prevent diverticulosis and lower the risk of colon cancer.

How Much Fibre Do You Need?

Your daily fibre requirements are tied to your calorie intake. That's why after age 50 when our calorie requirement declines, so does our fibre requirement.

Daily Fibre Requirements

	RDA (g)
Children, 1 to 3 years	19
Children, 4 to 8 years	25
Males, 9 to 13 years	31
Females, 9 to 18 years	26
Males, 14 to 50 years	38
Males, 50+ years	30
Females, 19 to 50 years	25
Females, 50+ years	21
During pregnancy	28
While breastfeeding	29

If you eat a 100 percent plant-based diet built on whole foods—which you will on *The Plant-Based Power Diet*—rest assured that you will get plenty of fibre each day. In fact, plant-based eaters can consume as much as 50 grams of fibre each day! Remember the plant-based daily menu I showed you on page 65 that supplied 67 grams of protein? Well, that menu provides 43 grams of fibre! This is in stark contrast to meat eaters, who get, on average, 14 grams of fibre per day—too little to reap fibre's health benefits.

Can Too Much Fibre Be Unhealthy?

There are some risks associated with consuming excessive fibre. Cramping, bloating and intestinal gas can occur. You might also become constipated if you don't drink enough water. That's because fibre needs water to be able to move through the intestinal tract. Very high intakes of fibre—50 grams or more per day—can also interfere with your intestine's ability to absorb minerals like calcium, magnesium, iron and zinc. But this effect is likely minimal and isn't a cause for concern. Plus, compared to refined foods, whole plant foods contain plenty of extra minerals to offset any losses.

To prevent the gastrointestinal side effects of a high-fibre diet, increase your fibre intake gradually over a period of three weeks. And be sure to drink plenty of water so fibre can work properly in the body. In Part 2, *The Plant-Based Power Diet*, you'll learn how much water you need to drink every day.

What About All the Gas?

While it's completely normal—and healthy—to produce gas, for some people it can be uncomfortable and embarrassing. Gas, or flatulence, occurs when bacteria that reside in your colon break down indigestible carbohydrates in plant foods. Culprits can be beans, lentils, soy foods, nuts, whole grains and cabbage family vegetables such as broccoli, Brussels sprouts, cabbage and cauliflower—pretty much all of the foods in a plant-based diet! The good news is that as your body adjusts to your new plant-based diet, so do those fermentation enzymes in your gut! Over time, gas becomes less of a problem for most people.

In the meantime, there are things you can do to minimize gas production. Start by eating smaller portions of problematic foods. If beans are a problem for you, eat lentils and split peas, which contain less gas-producing carbohydrates. You can also remove these carbohydrates by rinsing canned beans in running cool water before you use them. Soaking dried beans overnight before cooking them will also reduce gassy carbohydrates. Many of my clients find that taking a digestive enzyme supplement, called Beano®, prevents gas. Beano® digests the gas-producing carbohydrates for you. And it works for all gassy foods, not just beans.

DO CARBOHYDRATES MAKE YOU FAT?

Despite the fact that low-carbohydrate diets are passé, many people still fear carbs, thinking that eating them will prompt weight gain. I suppose that's the unfortunate legacy of the high-protein, Atkins-style diet era. Is there any truth to claims that high-carbohydrate diets can pack on the pounds? Yes and no. Sure, eating too much carbohydrate can make you fat, just like eating too much fat or too much protein can. But not *all* carbohydrates make you fat, nor do they increase your risk of health problems. What's most important is the *quality* of the carbohydrate-rich foods you eat.

Consider this fact: Populations around the world that eat a high-carbohydrate, low-fat diet enjoy the leanest body weights, not to mention the lowest rates of disease. Mediterranean, Asian and vegetarian diets all provide at least 55 percent of calories from carbohydrates from plant foods like grains, beans, fruit and vegetables. These high-carbohydrate diets differ considerably from the North American low-fat, high-carb diet that's built on convenience foods. The hallmark carbohydrate foods of the North American diet aren't legumes, fruit and vegetables. Instead, they're refined, processed carbs like low-fat cookies, fat-free cereal bars, baked tortilla chips, bagels and crackers that trigger hunger and promote weight gain.

A high-carb, low-fat plant-based diet is loaded with fibre, vitamins, minerals, antioxidants and protective plant chemicals, all of which can keep you healthy and trim. On the other hand, *refined* carbohydrates can affect your desire to continue eating, promote weight gain and raise your blood fats—and perhaps even increase your risk for heart disease, diabetes and cancer.

The Plant-Based Power Diet features high-quality carbs that will help keep you trim. And of course I'll give you a guide to choosing portion sizes that are right for you and your weight goal, be it to lose, maintain or put on a few extra pounds.

Low Glycemic: The Best Carbs to Eat

A whole foods, plant-based diet contains the healthiest carbohydrates around. Not only are these foods packed with fibre and nutrients, but the vast majority of whole plant foods have what's called a low glycemic index. That means they're digested slowly and, as a result, enter your bloodstream as glucose gradually. High glycemic foods like refined grains and sugary foods are digested more quickly and cause your blood glucose to spike. Why is this important? Because how quickly glucose enters your bloodstream can affect your hunger, your weight and your risk for diabetes and certain cancers.

When high glycemic carbohydrate foods spike your blood glucose, they cause an outpouring of insulin, the hormone that sends sugar from the blood to cells, where it's burned for energy. The end result is a low blood sugar level that can bring on hunger and fatigue. A steady intake of high glycemic index carbohydrates can also lead to insulin resistance, a condition that occurs when your cells can't properly respond to the action of insulin. Insulin resistance usually develops with obesity and heralds the onset of type 2 diabetes.

The glycemic index (GI) ranks foods by how fast they raise blood sugar levels using a scale of 0 to 100. All foods are compared to pure glucose, which is ranked 100. High glycemic foods (GI =70 or higher) include white bread, whole wheat bread, baked potatoes, refined breakfast cereals, instant oatmeal, cereal bars, Pop-Tarts, raisins, dates and table sugar.

Foods with a low GI (GI = less than 55) include grainy breads with seeds, steel-cut and large flake oats, 100% bran cereals, brown rice, quinoa, sweet potatoes, pasta, apples, berries, citrus fruit, grapes, pears, legumes, nuts and soy milk.

The Glycemic Index (GI) of Selected Plant Foods
Less than 55 = low GI; 55 to 70 = medium GI; greater than 70 = high GI

	GI value
Bread and crackers	
Pita bread, whole wheat	57
Pumpernickel, whole grain	51
Whole wheat bread	69
Breakfast cereals	
All-Bran, Kellogg's	51
All-Bran Buds with psyllium, Kellogg's	45
Bran Flakes	74
Corn Flakes	84
Oat Bran	50
Oatmeal, made from large flake oats	42
Raisin Bran	73
Shredded Wheat, spoon size	58
Special K	54
Pasta, grains and potato	
Barley	25
Bulgur	48
Corn	55
Couscous	65
Potato, new, unpeeled, boiled	62
Potato, red, skinned, mashed	91
Potato, red, skinned, boiled	88
Potato, white, skinned, baked	85
Potato, sweet, mashed	54
Rice, basmati	58
Rice, brown	55
Rice, converted, Uncle Ben's	44
Rice, long grain, white	56

	GI value
Spaghetti, whole wheat	37
Spaghetti, white	41
Legumes and soy	
Baked beans	48
Black beans	31
Black bean soup	64
Chickpeas, canned	42
Kidney beans	27
Lentils	30
Lentil soup, canned	34
Split pea soup	66
Soy beans	18
Soy beverage	31
Fruit	
Apple	38
Apricot, dried	31
Banana	51
Cantaloupe	65
Cherries	22
Dates, dried	103
Grapefruit	25
Grapes	46
Mango	55
Orange	44
Peach, canned	30
Pear	38
Raisins	64
Watermelon	72

	GI value
Sugars	
Agave syrup (nectar)	10–19
Fructose (fruit sugar)	23
Glucose	100
Honey	58
Lactose (milk sugar)	46
Sucrose (table sugar)	65

Source: Foster-Powell K and Brand Miller J. International tables of glycemic index. *American Journal of Clinical Nutrition* 62:871S–893S, 1995.

It's important to keep in mind that GI values are based on eating a single food on an empty stomach. The size of a meal and the variety of foods eaten together can skew the glycemic index. For instance, eating raisins (high GI) with a bowl of bran cereal (low GI) and soy milk (low GI) results in a meal that has a low to medium glycemic index.

Glycemic Index Versus Glycemic Load

The glycemic index tells you how quickly a particular food is converted to blood sugar, but it doesn't tell you how much carbohydrate is actually in that food. For instance, if you eat a serving of food that contains very little carbohydrate, it won't have much impact on your blood sugar and insulin level, regardless of its glycemic index.

That's where the glycemic load (GL) comes in. It's a concept that builds on the glycemic index to give a fuller picture of how a food or meal affects your blood glucose level. The GL takes into account a food's glycemic index *and* the grams of carbohydrate in the food or meal. Take watermelon, for example. It has a high GI, but because it doesn't have a lot of carbohydrate, its GL is relatively low. If you want to know the GI or GL of certain foods, I recommend that you visit www.glycemicindex.com. This website is updated regularly by researchers at the University of Sydney in Australia, the home of the glycemic index.

If this all sounds too complicated, not to worry. On *The Plant-Based Power Diet* you don't need a calculator, nor do you need to memorize a lengthy list of GI or GL values. Here's why: A whole foods, plant-based diet is optimal for blood sugar control! It's packed with fibre-rich, low glycemic foods that energize your body and keep your appetite in check.

What About Gluten? Should You Avoid It?

Have you noticed that gluten-free diets are becoming popular? In part, that's because gluten intolerance—or celiac disease—is on the rise. But they're also becoming fashionable as celebrities and professional athletes drop gluten from their diets. It's not uncommon to hear that switching to a gluten-free diet boosts energy, improves athletic performance and leads to weight loss. So what's the real deal? Is gluten—a protein found in wheat, rye and barley—something you should avoid? Or is a gluten-free diet simply the fad du jour?

Who does need a gluten-free diet? For starters, it's a necessity for people with celiac disease. One in 133 Canadians has celiac disease, a lifelong, genetically based disorder that occurs when the gluten protein triggers an abnormal immune response that injures the lining of the small intestine. This damage can interfere with the absorption of nutrients and cause symptoms such as diarrhea, abdominal pain, weight loss and, in children, delayed growth. But most people have symptoms that are more subtle, such as bloating, gas, fatigue or iron deficiency.

For people with celiac disease, following a gluten-free diet is the only way to treat the condition. The diet excludes obvious sources of gluten such as bread and pasta but also eliminates gluten that's hidden in many foods such as deli meats, salad dressings and condiments.

Eating gluten can also cause symptoms in people who don't have celiac disease. People who have what's called non-celiac gluten sensitivity test negative for celiac disease but react poorly to gluten and often complain of abdominal pain, headaches and fatigue. They feel much better when eating a gluten-free diet.

So what about the rest of us? Is it a good idea to give up gluten and avoid pasta, bread, crackers and hundreds of other foods? No. There's not a stitch of evidence that following a gluten-free diet will promote weight loss or offer any health benefit beyond helping gluten-sensitive people.

However, if you do decide to drop gluten from your diet, be sure to include gluten-free whole grains such as brown and wild rice, quinoa and millet to help you get fibre, vitamins, minerals and antioxidants. Too often I see people filling up on gluten-free bread, bagels, crackers and cookies made from refined flours that have been stripped of fibre and nutrients. And unlike wheat flour, they are not enriched with vitamins and minerals. Many gluten-free packaged foods are also higher in carbohydrates and sodium.

Keep in mind that gluten-free diets tend to be low in fibre because wheat bran—a major source of fibre—is off limits. To add fibre, include 2 tablespoons of ground flaxseed in your daily diet. Legumes and lentils are also high-fibre foods appropriate for a gluten-free diet. Eating at least three fruit servings and four vegetable servings every day will boost your fibre intake, too. *The Plant-Based Power Diet* will help you eat a fibre- and nutrient-rich gluten-free diet.

Quick Tips for Choosing Healthy Carbs

• Limit refined, added sugars in your diet. (A whole foods, plant-based diet is low in sugar, so this shouldn't be a problem!) Read ingredient lists on packaged foods to choose foods that contain few—or no—added sugars.
• Most often, choose whole grains like brown rice, quinoa, millet, whole wheat couscous, hulled barley and whole wheat or brown rice pasta. Choose breads and cereals that are 100% whole grain.
• Eat a variety of plant-based foods every day to get good sources of soluble and insoluble fibre in your diet. Excellent sources of soluble fibre include oats, oat bran, barley and okra. Wheat bran, 100% whole wheat products and nuts contain mainly insoluble fibre.

- If gas is a problem, consider using a digestive enzyme supplement like Beano® to break down carbohydrates in legumes and other foods that our bodies can't digest.
- Include at least two low glycemic foods at every meal. Again, this is not hard to do on a whole foods, plant-based diet since legumes, soy, nuts and many whole grains and fruits release their carbohydrate slowly—rather than quickly—into your bloodstream.

Include the Right Balance of Healthy Fats

Plant-based diets tend to be lower in fat than the average North American diet since they don't include meat, dairy and eggs. The biggest difference, however, in a diet that is centred on plant foods rather than animal foods is the type of fat it contains. Unlike a meat-based diet that can be laden with saturated fat, it's pretty difficult to find unhealthy fats in a plant-based diet. But there's more to a healthy plant-based diet than low saturated fat. As you'll soon learn, it's also important to get the right balance of certain fats in your diet. Before I tell you how much and what types of fat to get in your plant-based diet, let's review the basics of dietary fat.

DIETARY FAT 101

Believe it or not, you do need to get some fat in your diet every day. Dietary fat supplies fat-soluble vitamins A, D, E and K, nutrients your body can't live without. Fat also provides certain fatty acids that are essential for health but that the body can't make on its own. You'll learn more about these *essential fatty acids* later in this section. Here's a primer on the different types of fat found in foods.

Saturated Fats

You won't find much saturated fat in *The Plant-Based Power Diet*. That's because it's found mainly in animal foods like meat, dairy and eggs. A diet high in saturated fat raises LDL, or bad, blood cholesterol. Having high LDL cholesterol can increase your risk of heart disease because it's linked to the process of hardening and narrowing of the arteries. Current guidelines recommend that we limit saturated fat as much as possible. But there's no need to worry about avoiding saturated fat since plant-based diets contain very, very little of it.

There is one potential source of saturated fat in a plant-based diet, however. Tropical plant oils such as coconut, palm and palm kernel oils contain saturated fat. Coconut oil, for instance, is nearly 90 percent saturated fat—more than butter (at 64 percent)! You'll find palm and palm kernel oil on the ingredient lists of many processed foods. You don't need to be concerned about tropical oils since a whole foods, plant-based diet discourages processed, packaged foods.

WHAT'S THE DEAL WITH COCONUT OIL?
You may have noticed that coconut oil is catching on these days. Perhaps you've even heard that coconut oil is the healthiest oil to cook with. I don't agree, but coconut oil isn't as bad as its high saturated fat content may make you think. The type of saturated fat in coconut (and palm) oil does raise total blood cholesterol, but it mainly boosts "good" HDL cholesterol. (HDL is called good because it's cholesterol that's moving away from your arteries to your liver to be broken down and removed from the body. Unlike LDL cholesterol, the HDL version doesn't build up on artery walls.) Even so, I don't recommend cooking everything in coconut oil since there are other oils that are healthier for your heart. And as you'll soon read, many gurus of plant-based nutrition advise against using any processed oils.

Trans Fats
Trans fats are formed during partial hydrogenation, a food industry process that hardens and stabilizes liquid vegetable oils, increasing their shelf life. Trans fats are added to commercial baked goods like cookies, cakes, pies and pastries, snack foods and some brands of margarine. French fries, onion rings, chicken nuggets and other deep-fried restaurant foods may also contain trans fats.

Trans fats are the worst type of fat for your health. A steady intake not only raises your LDL cholesterol, but also decreases your good HDL cholesterol. Eating too much has also been tied to a greater risk of type 2 diabetes. It's nasty stuff. That's why we're advised to keep our trans fat intake as low as possible—there is no safe level! That's not hard to do on a whole foods, plant-based diet! If you do buy packaged foods on occasion, read the nutrition labels to select foods that don't contain any trans fat. Foods with a Daily Value (DV) of 10 percent or less for saturated plus trans fat are considered low in these two fats.

Monounsaturated Fats

This family of fats has been considered heart healthy ever since researchers linked higher intakes of monounsaturated fats with lower death rates from heart disease. Since then, we've learned that monounsaturated fats can raise HDL cholesterol. These fats may also help reduce inflammation in the body. What's more, studies conducted in people with diabetes have found that monounsaturated fats can improve how the body uses the sugar-clearing hormone insulin.

Where can you get monounsaturated fats in your diet? Olive oil, canola oil, peanut oil, high oleic sunflower and safflower oil, avocado, most nuts (except for walnuts), nut butters and olives are all good sources.

Polyunsaturated Fats

Polyunsaturated fats are found in oily fish like salmon, trout and sardines, vegetable oils, nuts and seeds. Corn, soybean, grapeseed, sunflower and safflower oils are rich sources of polyunsaturated fats, or polys for short. Polys are considered good fats because they have a number of health benefits when they replace saturated fats in the diet. They can lower LDL cholesterol while increasing HDL cholesterol. They can also help combat inflammation in the body.

ESSENTIAL FATTY ACIDS: A BALANCING ACT

Polyunsaturated fats also provide essential fatty acids (EFAs) called linoleic acid (an omega-6 fatty acid) and alpha-linolenic acid (an omega-3 fatty acid). EFAs help form cell membranes, maintain

Omega what?

A fatty acid is a long chain of carbons bonded together, which are in turn bonded to many hydrogens. If all of the bonds between the carbons are single bonds, the fatty acid is classified as saturated. If a fatty acid has one double bond between two carbons, it's monounsaturated. Polyunsaturated fatty acids have two or more double bonds.

Scientists use the Greek omega system to indicate where a double bond is located on a fatty acid. For example, omega-3 fatty acids have their first double bond located three carbons away from the end; the first double bond of omega-6 fatty acids is located six carbons away. Why am I telling you this? Because the location of these double bonds makes a big difference to how fatty acids are metabolized by your body and, as you'll read below, how they affect your health.

a healthy immune system, keep our vision sharp and produce compounds called eicosanoids. They're essential because our bodies can't make them on their own so they must be supplied by our diet. And because linoleic acid (LA) and alpha-linolenic acid (ALA) are essential to our health, we have daily requirements for each just as we do for vitamins and minerals.

Getting the right balance of EFAs in your diet is important for optimal health. Omega-6 fatty acids are used to produce eicosanoids—hormone-like compounds—that promote inflammation and increase blood pressure and blood clotting. (You'll recall from Step 1 that ongoing inflammation is a powerful contributor to many chronic diseases.) More omega-3s and fewer omega-6s, on the other hand, favour the formation of eicosanoids that protect against these effects. The body uses omega-3 fatty acids to make anti-inflammatory compounds that support good health.

It's important to have the right balance of omega-6s and omega-3s because each type of fat competes for the same enzymes that are needed to transform them into either inflammatory or anti-inflammatory eicosanoids. If you have plenty of omega-6 fatty acids and few omega-3 fatty acids in your diet, the harmful eicosanoids will win out. On the flip side, if your diet is plentiful in omega-3s and limits omega-6s, the body will make more anti-inflammatory compounds.

The problem is that our modern diet is overwhelmed by omega-6 linoleic acid from vegetable oils in processed and fast foods. Add to this the fact that most of us eat too few omega-3 fats. Even some fish eaters consume too few omega-3 fatty acids for optimal health. Plant-based eaters can consume even less since they don't eat fish. Fish and seafood contain two omega-3 fats called DHA (docosahexaenoic acid) and EPA (eicosapentaenoic acid).

Experts estimate that our current diet provides up to 20 times more omega-6s than omega-3s, a ratio that can undermine our health. The ideal ratio of omega-6s to omega-3s is somewhere between 2:1 and 4:1. That means you should consume only two to four times as much omega-6 as omega-3 fats. I'll tell you how to increase your intake of plant-based omega-3s later in this step.

Cholesterol

This waxy, fatty substance is used by the body to make important hormones, vitamin D and bile acids, which help digest the fat in a meal. But there's no need for any cholesterol in the diet since your body can make all it needs on its own. That's why, unlike vitamins and minerals, there isn't a daily requirement for cholesterol.

Consuming too much cholesterol from foods can increase LDL blood cholesterol. But people vary considerably in their response, probably because of genetic factors. Some research suggests that people with diabetes may absorb more cholesterol from foods and, as a result, are more responsive to its blood cholesterol–raising effect. We're advised to limit our cholesterol intake to less than 300 milligrams per day. If you have heart disease, your daily cholesterol intake should not exceed 200 milligrams per day.

Cholesterol comes almost exclusively from animal foods. Rich sources include liver, egg yolks, shrimp, lobster, fatty cuts of meat and high-fat dairy products such as cream, butter and cheese. You'll be consuming virtually no cholesterol on *The Plant-Based Power Diet*.

HOW MUCH FAT SHOULD YOU EAT?

It's a million-dollar question and one that's hotly debated: What's the ideal fat intake in a plant-based diet? There are two schools of thought in the world of plant-based nutrition. In one camp are the proponents of a very low–fat, plant-based diet that gets no more than 10 percent of its calories from fat. That's much less than our national guidelines, which advise eating a diet with 20 to 35 percent fat. Eating more than this amount of fat, especially the wrong type of fat, can promote excess weight gain, obesity and chronic disease. Consuming less could rob your body of fat-soluble vitamins A, D, E and K. Champions of a very low-fat diet advise against the use of cooking oils and high-fat plant foods such as olives, avocado and nuts and seeds.

The Evidence for Low Fat

There are data to support a 10 percent fat plant-based diet. Dr. Caldwell B. Esselstyn Jr., the Cleveland Clinic doctor I introduced you to in Step 2, used such a diet to reverse heart disease in his patients. After 12 years on a plant-based diet, 70 percent of Dr. Esselstyn's patients experienced a measureable reversal of their heart disease. Dr. Dean Ornish, a renowned American physician who has authored a number of books, also used a low-fat diet to treat heart patients. In fact, Dr. Ornish was the first medical doctor to provide documented proof that a very low-fat, plant-based diet—in combination with lifestyle changes—could bring about the regression of blocked coronary arteries. Patients on his program experienced near complete relief from their chest pain while patients in the control group had their atherosclerosis (hardening and narrowing of the arteries) progress.

The Evidence for Moderate—but Good—Fat

Other experts believe that it's the quality, rather than the quantity, of fat you eat that's most important for health. This notion stemmed from 1960s research called the Seven Countries Study, which linked the dietary habits of people living in different countries to rates of heart disease. Surprisingly, the lowest rates of dying from heart disease weren't found in countries where a low-fat diet was consumed. Instead, the high-fat Greek diet was the heart healthiest. On the Greek island of Crete, rates of chronic diseases were among the lowest in the world and life expectancy was the highest. Residents of the island ate a primarily plant-based diet that was low in saturated fat and cholesterol and high in monounsaturated fat.

More proof that the type of fat, rather than the amount of fat, could be a more important predictor of heart health came decades later. The Lyon Diet Heart Study tested a Mediterranean-style diet in heart attack patients to see if it could prevent future heart problems. The diet was based on fruits, vegetables, grains, beans and fish and included canola-oil margarine as its fat source (canola oil is rich in monounsaturated fat). After nearly four years on the diet, patients were 72 percent less likely than control patients to suffer a second heart attack or die from heart disease.[1]

A Mediterranean-style diet, rich in monounsaturated fat, has been shown to help guard against heart disease as well as certain cancers, obesity, diabetes, asthma, Parkinson's disease and Alzheimer's disease. And it's been shown to increase life expectancy.

What's the Right Amount of Fat?

By now you may be wondering who's right. While these views seem to contradict one another, they actually have more in common than you might think. A low-fat, plant-based diet and the Mediterranean-style diet both feature fruits, vegetables, grains, legumes and other plant foods packed with fibre, vitamins, minerals and disease-fighting phytochemicals. In fact, scientists speculate that the Mediterranean-style diet's health benefits are due to its strong antioxidant and anti-inflammatory effects. Both diets are low in unhealthy fats.

Both diets don't contain much linoleic acid, either. A very low-fat, whole foods, plant-based diet doesn't include any added oils. And olive oil, the main source of fat in the Mediterranean-style diet, is very low in linoleic acid. (Remember that linoleic acid is an omega-6 fatty acid found in polyunsaturated oils like corn, grapeseed, soybean, sunflower and safflower.)

I don't think it's necessary to drastically cut fat on a plant-based diet. There's no research to show that a plant-based diet that includes a moderate amount of healthy fat harms your health. Rather, research suggests the very opposite. In my opinion, what's important is that you eat a variety of whole plant foods every day while keeping saturated fat, cholesterol and refined starches and sugars to a minimum. *The Plant-Based Power Diet* helps you do just that. It also allows you to eat a moderate amount of healthy fats from whole foods like avocados, nuts, seeds and olives—foods that also provide valuable nutrients. And if you like, you can also use a little olive oil or canola oil. But if you'd rather stick to a 10 percent fat version of *The Plant-Based Power Diet*, that's fine, too. You'll find a meal plan that allows you to choose the amount of fat that's right for you.

HOW TO GET YOUR OMEGA-3s

I told you earlier that it's important to have the right balance of omega-3s and omega-6s. Your diet should provide enough omega-3 fats and not too many omega-6 fats. Studies have found that a higher intake of DHA and EPA, the two omega-3 fats found in fish and seafood, helps protect from heart disease, heart attack, macular degeneration, arthritis, Alzheimer's disease, depression and possibly some types of cancers. DHA is also critical during pregnancy and breastfeeding for a baby's normal brain development and vision.

ALA: A Plant-Based Omega-3 Fatty Acid

Since a plant-based diet doesn't include fish, is it possible to get omega-3 fats? Can you get enough of these healthy fats from plant foods? Remember alpha-linolenic acid (ALA)? Well, this omega-3 fatty acid is found only in plant foods! It's plentiful in flaxseeds, chia seeds, hemp seeds, walnuts, soybeans and soy products. Canola oil contains some ALA, too. It's also added to some brands of soy beverages. Once consumed, some ALA is converted to EPA, which is then converted to DHA. It's DHA that has the most potent health benefits in the body.

Unfortunately, our bodies are unable to convert very much ALA to EPA and DHA. To maximize this conversion, you need to include good sources of ALA in your diet every day. It's also very important to minimize your intake of omega-6 fatty acids, which compete with omega-3s for conversion to eicosanoids. If you do use cooking oil, use monounsaturated oils like olive and canola since these are low in linoleic acid. Because ALA is considered an "essential" fatty acid, a daily Adequate Intake level has been set. Here's how much ALA you need to consume every day.

How Much Alpha-Linolenic Acid (ALA) Do You Need?

	Daily Adequate Intake (g)
Children, 1 to 3 years	0.7
Children, 4 to 8 years	0.9
Males, 9 to 13 years	1.2
Females, 9 to 13 years	1.0
Males, 14+ years	1.6
Females, 14+ years	1.1
During pregnancy	1.4
While breastfeeding	1.3

To maximize conversion of ALA to EPA, some experts recommend that plant-based eaters consume much more than the recommended intake—at least 4 grams of ALA each day. As you'll see on page 96, there are plenty of plant foods to help you reach your daily ALA target.

Alpha-Linolenic Acid (ALA) in Plant Foods

	ALA content (g)
Avocado, 1/2	0.1
Broccoli, cooked, 1 cup (250 mL)	0.2
Canola oil, 1 tbsp (15 mL)	1.3
Chia seeds, ground, 1 tbsp (15 mL)	2.1
Chia seeds, whole, 1 tbsp (15 mL)	1.8
Collard greens, cooked, 1 cup (250 mL)	0.2
Flaxseed oil, 1 tbsp (15 g)	7.2
Flaxseed oil supplement, 1 capsule (1 g)	0.5
Flaxseed, ground	1.6
Flaxseed, shelled (e.g., Omega Crunch), 1 tbsp (15 mL)	2.2
Hemp beverage, 1 cup (250 mL)	1.0
Hemp butter, 1 tbsp (15 mL)	1.2
Hemp hearts, 1 tbsp (15 mL)	0.8
Hempseed oil, 1 tbsp (15 mL)	2.0
Kale, cooked, 1 cup (250 mL)	0.1
Pecan halves, 1/4 cup (50 mL)	0.5
Soybeans, cooked, 1/2 cup (125 mL)	0.5
Soybeans, edamame, shelled, 1/2 cup (125 mL)	0.3
Soy beverage, 1 cup (250 mL)	0.2
Soy nuts, 1/4 cup (50 mL)	0.7
Tempeh, 1/2 cup (125 mL)	0.2
Tofu, firm, 1/2 cup (125 mL)	0.2
Walnuts, shelled, 1/4 cup (50 mL)	2.2
Walnut oil, 1 tbsp (15 mL)	1.4

Getting DHA from Plants, Not Fish

Provided you're getting enough ALA every day—and you're not consuming too much omega-6 linoleic acid—your body will be able to convert more ALA to EPA. However, research suggests that supplementing your diet with ALA doesn't increase the level of DHA in the blood.[2] It is DHA, not EPA, that's so important for the proper functioning of your brain as an adult and for the development of your brain and visual abilities during the first six months of life.

For this reason, it's a good idea to get a direct source of DHA from a supplement or DHA-fortified foods. Vegetarian DHA supplements made from algae are available to help you increase your intake of omega-3 fats. Research shows that taking DHA supplements can markedly raise blood DHA levels in vegans.[3] Take 200 to 400 milligrams per day. (Fish are actually the intermediary when it comes to delivering DHA. They get their DHA by eating microscopic algae, which produce it.)

You can also buy food products fortified with vegetarian DHA to help you increase your intake. So Good Omega DHA soy beverage, for example, contains 32 milligrams of DHA per 1 cup (250 mL) serving. DHA algae oil is also added to Canada Bread's Smart Bread, which contains 0.1 gram (100 milligrams) of omega-3 per two slices.

Quick Tips for Choosing the Right Fats
- Keep your fat intake to 20 to 35 percent of daily calories, or 20 to 35 grams of fat for every 1000 calories. To follow a very low-fat, plant-based diet, keep fat intake to 10 percent of daily calories, about 10 grams of fat per 1000 calories.
- Get most of your fat from whole foods such as avocado, nuts, seeds and olives that also supply vitamins, minerals and phytochemicals.
- Limit your intake of oils that contain a high amount of omega-6 linoleic acid, including corn, soybean, grapeseed, sunflower and safflower oils. Read labels on food packages to avoid foods that list these oils as one of the first few ingredients.
- Include good sources of omega-3 alpha-linolenic acid (ALA) in your diet every day. These include flaxseed and flax oil, chia seeds, hemp seeds, walnuts, soybeans and soy foods.
- Supplement your diet with DHA derived from algae. Take 200 to 400 milligrams per day.

Find Your Calcium in Non-Dairy Sources

We've been programmed for years to believe that eating dairy products is the only way to get enough calcium for strong bones. It is true that milk, yogurt and cheese are exceptional sources of calcium. But they're not the only foods that deliver plenty of this bone-building mineral. Believe it or not, there are many plant foods that contain substantial amounts of calcium. In fact, it's entirely possible to meet your daily calcium requirements with a plant-based diet—without taking a supplement! And if you take dietary measures to prevent losing calcium from your body, you're well on your way to keeping your bones strong by eating a diet void of cow's milk.

CALCIUM FOR HEALTHY BONES

The fact that almost all—99 percent—of our body's calcium is housed within our skeleton and teeth underlines its importance to bone health. The remaining calcium circulates in our blood-stream, where it's used for critical functions such as conducting nerve impulses, regulating your heartbeat, contracting muscles and forming blood clots. Your body tightly controls the level of blood calcium, so measuring it doesn't give you a picture of your body's calcium status. Instead, the density of your bones does.

Your bones are constantly being broken down and rebuilt. During the bone-building process, cells secrete bone mineral made up of calcium and phosphorus. It's this mineral complex that gives bones their strength and rigidity. Until our late twenties, we build more bone than we lose. Then, we start to lose more bone than we build up naturally as we age. This is especially true for women during the early post-menopausal years, who lose bone at a much faster rate than men. Losing too much calcium causes bones to become weak, increasing the risk of osteoporosis.

When your diet is low in calcium and your blood-calcium level falls too low, hormones go to work to bring calcium back to your bloodstream. Some of this calcium comes from your bones—it's removed from your skeleton to rebalance your blood calcium. The bottom line: When you shortchange your diet, you shortchange your bones, too. That's why a calcium-rich diet is necessary to keep your body's calcium stores well balanced and your bones strong.

Preventing Calcium Loss:
The Protein, Sodium, Caffeine and Soft Drink Connection

There's more to healthy bones than getting enough calcium in your plant-based diet. It's also vital to ensure that you aren't eating certain foods that can cause excess calcium to be excreted from your body. A diet too high in protein—especially animal protein—causes more calcium to be lost in the urine. That's because sulphur-containing amino acids in animal-protein foods make the blood more acidic. When this happens, your body releases calcium from your bones to neutralize this acid. A plant-based diet is more alkaline (the opposite of acidic) than a meat-based diet and, as a result, helps maintain the density of your bones. But it's still important to not overeat protein. Even plant foods contain sulphur-containing amino acids, although much less than do meat, eggs and dairy. Even so, the effect of eating too much protein is likely more pronounced in people who don't meet daily calcium requirements. In fact, protein appears to be beneficial to bone health in people who get more calcium in their diet.

It's also important to watch your sodium intake since too much sodium increases calcium excretion. Adults aged 19 to 50 need only 1500 milligrams of sodium each day and older adults need only 1300 milligrams. (The safe upper limit for sodium is 2300 milligrams per day.) Yet most North Americans consume twice as much thanks to our penchant for processed foods and restaurant meals.

To keep sodium within recommended limits, stay clear of the salt shaker, minimize the use of salt in cooking and choose packaged foods that are low in added salt. Read nutrition labels: Foods with a daily value for sodium of 5 percent or less are low in this mineral. But that doesn't mean you can't eat a food that's higher in sodium. Just be sure to balance your sodium intake over the course of the day. The good news is that you don't have to worry about consuming excessive sodium on a plant-based diet centred on whole, unprocessed foods.

Caffeine and phosphoric acid, an additive in cola drinks (both regular and diet), can leach calcium from your bones, too. Aim to consume at most 400 milligrams of caffeine per day, the amount found in three 8-ounce cups of coffee. If you have low bone mass or osteoporosis, limit your daily caffeine intake to 200 milligrams, about one 8-ounce cup of coffee. As for soft drinks, I don't recommend them, not even sugar-free versions. You're much better off drinking water or calcium-fortified beverages.

HOW MUCH CALCIUM DO YOU NEED?

Ensuring that your diet provides enough calcium each day is necessary to help minimize losses of the mineral and maintain the density of your bones. While one study found plant-based eaters to have worse bone health than meat eaters, this was because they had lower calcium intakes. When calcium was plentiful in the diet, the risk of bone fracture was the same between plant-based eaters and meat eaters. Here's how much calcium you need each day; the recommended daily intakes are the same as those for people who eat dairy products.

Recommended Dietary Allowances (RDAs) for Calcium

	Calcium (mg)
Children, 1 to 3 years	700
Children, 4 to 8 years	1000
Boys and girls, 9 to 18 years	1300
Females, 19 to 50 years	1000
Males, 19 to 70 years	1000
Females, 50+ years	1200
Males, 70+ years	1200

While it's essential to get enough calcium in your diet each day, it's also important to not consume too much. A very high intake of calcium can cause kidney stones and kidney problems. It can also prevent your body from properly absorbing other minerals such as iron, zinc and phosphorus. How much calcium is too much? The safe upper daily limit for calcium from food and supplements combined—an amount you should not exceed—is as follows.

Safe Upper Limits for Daily Calcium Intake

	Calcium (mg)
Children, 1 to 8 years	2500
Boys and girls, 9 to 18 years	3000
Males and females, 19 to 50 years	2500
Males and females, 50+ years	2000

MINING FOR CALCIUM IN A PLANT-BASED DIET

The plant kingdom is full of foods rich in calcium. After all, that's where cows get their calcium—by eating grass and other plants that have absorbed the mineral from the ground. In a plant-based diet you'll find calcium in fortified plant beverages and juices, calcium-set tofu (look for calcium sulphate on the ingredient list), legumes, nuts and leafy green vegetables. Even mineral water adds calcium to your diet.

In order for foods to be good sources of calcium, the mineral needs to be in a form that your body can absorb. This is called *bioavailable* calcium and it's the calcium your body can use. So even if a food boasts plenty of calcium, this doesn't mean your body will absorb all of it. Some plant foods contain oxalates and phytates, natural compounds that bind to calcium, causing calcium to be poorly absorbed. Leafy greens such as Swiss chard, spinach, beet greens and rhubarb contain a lot of oxalate, limiting the amount of calcium available to your body. For instance, only 5 percent of the total calcium in spinach is bioavailable, compared to 31 percent in soy milk.[1] Much of the calcium in nuts, pinto beans and kidney beans is bound up with oxalates.

Fortunately, there are many plant foods that contain highly bioavailable calcium. Broccoli, Brussels sprouts, bok choy, cabbage, cauliflower, kale, collard greens, turnip greens and turnips all deliver calcium that's well absorbed by your body. As do fortified soy milk and other calcium-enriched beverages. The following tips will help you add plant foods, plentiful in bioavailable calcium, to your daily diet.

Quick Tips to Enhance Calcium Absorption

- Enjoy your greens cooked more often than raw. Cooking boosts the bioavailable calcium by releasing what's bound to oxalates and phytates.
- Keep iron and calcium supplements separate. Iron and calcium compete with each other for absorption in the gut. If you take iron supplements to treat an iron deficiency, do not take them with a calcium-rich meal.
- Drink tea between, rather than during, meals. Tannins, natural compounds in tea, inhibit calcium absorption.
- Make sure you're meeting daily requirements for vitamin D. This nutrient helps you absorb calcium from foods. (You'll learn how much vitamin D you need—and how to get it—in Step 8.)

Calcium Content of Plant Foods

	Calcium (mg)
Calcium-fortified plant and fruit beverages	
Almond milk, 1 cup (250 mL)	300 to 330
Hemp milk, 1 cup (250 mL)	300 to 330
Oat milk, 1 cup (250 mL)	300 to 350
Rice milk, 1 cup (250 mL)	300 to 330
Soy milk, 1 cup (250 mL)	300 to 330
Orange juice, 1 cup (250 mL)	300 to 360
Legumes and soy	
Baked beans, 1 cup (250 mL)	154
Black beans, 1 cup (250 mL)	84
Garbanzo beans (chickpeas), 1 cup (250 mL)	65
Kidney beans, 1 cup, cooked (250 mL)	92
Lentils, cooked, 1 cup (250 mL)	38
Lima beans, cooked, 1 cup (250 mL)	54
Navy beans, cooked, 1 cup (250 mL)	123
Pinto beans, cooked, 1 cup (250 mL)	175
Soybeans, cooked, 1 cup (250 mL)	261
Soy nuts, roasted, 1/4 cup (50 mL)	60
Tempeh, cooked, 3 1/2 ounces (100 g)	96
Tofu, raw, firm, with calcium sulphate, 1/2 cup (125 mL)	253
Nuts and seeds and nut butters	
Almonds, whole, 1/4 cup (50 mL)	94
Almond butter, 2 tbsp (25 mL)	112
Brazil nuts, 1/4 cup (50 mL)	53
Peanuts, 1/4 cup (50 mL)	34
Peanut butter, 2 tbsp (25 mL)	14
Sunflower seeds, 1/4 cup (50 mL)	22

	Calcium (mg)
Vegetables	
Cabbage, cooked, 1 cup (250 mL)	72
Beet greens, cooked, 1 cup (250 mL)	164
Bok choy, cooked, 1 cup (250 mL)	158
Broccoli, raw, 1 cup (250 mL)	42
Broccoli, cooked, 1 cup (250 mL)	62
Brussels sprouts, cooked, 1 cup (250 mL)	56
Collard greens, cooked, 1 cup (250 mL)	266
Kale, cooked, 1 cup (250 mL)	94
Okra, cooked, 1 cup (250 mL)	124
Rapini (Broccoli raab), cooked, 1 cup (250 mL)	200
Spinach, cooked, 1 cup (250 mL)	245
Spinach, frozen, cooked, 1 cup (250 mL)	290
Swiss chard, cooked, 1 cup (250 mL)	102
Turnip, cooked, 1 cup (250 mL)	76
Turnip greens, cooked, 1 cup (250 mL)	197
Other foods	
Figs, dried, 5	68
Orange, 1 medium	66
Blackstrap molasses, 1 tbsp (15 mL)	180

Source: USDA Agricultural Research Service. National Agricultural Library. National Nutrient Database for Standard Reference, Release 25. 2012.

DO YOU NEED A CALCIUM SUPPLEMENT?

It's possible to meet your daily calcium requirement, but it does take some planning. Even people who drink milk and eat yogurt need to pay attention to calcium since many don't meet daily calcium targets. You'll find it much easier to get enough calcium if you use fortified plant beverages. But you also need to include a variety of calcium-rich plant foods in your diet each day. Take a look at the meal plan on page 65, Step 4. The inclusion of soy milk, calcium-set tofu, chickpeas, almonds and cooked broccoli helped bring daily calcium to 1199 milligrams! *The Plant-Based Power Diet* in Part 2 guides you on how many calcium-rich foods to include in your diet each day.

That being said, some people may need to take a calcium supplement to meet daily needs. Older adults, who need more calcium for bone health, may need to bridge the gap in their diet with a supplement. If you'd like to lose a little weight and decide to follow a lower-calorie meal plan on *The Plant-Based Power Diet*, you also may benefit from a supplement. I'll guide you on whether a supplement is necessary for your meal plan.

You can't rely on a multivitamin and mineral supplement to provide enough calcium since most brands contain 100 to 125 milligrams of the mineral. Which calcium product you choose will depend on convenience, absorbability and tolerance.

Calcium Carbonate versus Calcium Citrate

The most common compounds used in calcium supplements are carbonate and citrate. These two compounds are attached to calcium in a supplement. Calcium carbonate supplements are generally the least expensive and most widely used. They typically contain twice as much elemental calcium—usually 500 or 600 milligrams per tablet—as supplements made from calcium citrate. Calcium citrate supplements contain between 250 and 350 milligrams of elemental calcium.

Elemental calcium is the amount of calcium in a supplement that's available for your body to absorb; it's the amount on which your daily calcium requirements are based. Most products list the amount of elemental calcium on the label. But some brands list only the total weight (in milligrams) of the tablet. This is the weight of the calcium plus the compound it's bound to: carbonate or citrate.

If you need to take 600 milligrams of calcium from a supplement, a calcium carbonate product may be more convenient. That's because you'd have to take more calcium citrate pills to get the same amount of elemental calcium as you'd get from a calcium carbonate pill.

But there are advantages to taking calcium citrate supplements. Calcium carbonate requires extra stomach acid for absorption so it's best taken with food or immediately after eating. Calcium carbonate wouldn't be the best choice if you're taking a medication that prevents your stomach from secreting acid. Calcium citrate, on the other hand, is readily absorbed so it can be taken any time of day, even on an empty stomach. I also like calcium citrate supplements because they provide pretty much the same amount of calcium that's found in a serving of fortified plant beverage.

If you do need to take a calcium supplement, spread your intake over the course of the day. Calcium absorption is best in a 500-milligram dose or less. That's because the more calcium you consume beyond 500 milligrams, the less your body absorbs. In other words, don't take your calcium supplement with a glass of soy milk that's rich in calcium. If you take medications, check with your pharmacist about possible interactions with calcium. Calcium can interfere with the body's ability to use certain drugs, including tetracycline, bisphosphonates (Fosamax, Actonel), hypothyroid medication (Synthroid) and iron supplements.

Calcium Supplements and Your Heart

All that being said about calcium supplements, I advise all of my clients—meat eaters and plant-based eaters—to try to get their calcium from foods first. That's because calcium-rich foods also supply many other nutrients and phytochemicals that are missing in supplements. As well, there's some concern that calcium supplements may not be as safe as we once thought.

Two recent analyses, in 2010 and 2011, sparked warnings that calcium supplements may increase the risk of heart attack. In 2010, New Zealand researchers reviewed 11 trials—none of them designed to assess heart attack risk—and concluded that older women who take calcium supplements have a 30 percent higher risk of heart attack. The actual number of heart attacks was small, though. Overall, 2.7 percent of women taking calcium pills had heart attacks compared with 2.2 percent taking placebo

(163 versus 130 heart attacks). The risk was greater in women who consumed more than 800 milligrams of calcium from their diet *and* took supplements, therefore exceeding the recommended daily intake.[2]

In 2011, the same researchers looked at data from a large study on women and calcium and vitamin D consumption and found that calcium plus vitamin D supplements raised the odds of heart attack by 24 percent.[3] It's thought that calcium supplements, especially in large doses, cause a rapid spike in blood calcium levels that could make its way to artery walls, causing them to stiffen and narrow.

The bottom line: These studies don't provide definitive proof that calcium supplements cause heart attacks. There's also no iron-clad evidence that calcium pills don't harm the heart. It's possible that calcium supplements may have a different effect in people who have some degree of coronary artery disease. In my opinion, the recent findings suggest there may be a downside from getting your calcium mainly or exclusively from supplements.

So, what to do? Do you need to be worried about taking a calcium supplement? If you are free of heart disease, you get *most* of your calcium from foods and you do not exceed your daily recommended calcium intake, it is fine to get some of your calcium from a supplement. If you need to bridge a gap in your diet, subtract the calcium you're getting from food from your 1000- or 1200-milligram calcium requirement. Supplement only up to that level. You don't need more.

Quick Tips for Getting Calcium in a Plant-Based Diet
- Use a calcium-fortified plant beverage like soy, rice, almond, oat or hemp milk, as these provide a good 300 milligrams of calcium per serving. (Keep in mind that only soy milk is a good source of protein.)
- When buying tofu, buy a product that's been processed with calcium. Look for calcium sulphate on the ingredient list.

- Include cooked green vegetables in your diet every day. Veggies with well-absorbed calcium—they're low in oxalates—include broccoli, Brussels sprouts, bok choy, kale, collard greens, rapini and turnip greens.
- Choose calcium-rich snacks such as soy nuts, edamame (young, green soybeans), almonds, almond butter and figs.
- If you drink orange juice, choose a calcium-fortified brand.
- Use *The Plant-Based Power Diet* meal plans on pages 151–152 to ensure you get enough calcium in your daily diet.

Step 8

Maximize Your Nutrients with a Wide Mix of Plant Foods

The key to a plant-based diet is variety. Eat a wide mix of plant foods—and meet your daily calorie requirements—and you'll get all of your vitamins and minerals in adequate amounts. That being said, there's some concern that 100 percent plant-based diets fall short where certain nutrients are concerned. Vitamin B_{12}, for example, occurs naturally only in animal foods. So it's crucial to include fortified foods in your diet or take a supplement. Iron, which is well absorbed from meat but not from plant foods, may also fall short in a plant-based diet. But knowing which nutrients you need to pay attention to, how much you need and what foods provide the most will ensure that your plant-based diet delivers optimal amounts of everything your body needs.

VITAL VITAMINS

Your body needs a daily supply of vitamins since it can't make them on its own. They're needed for normal growth and to keep your body's tissues and cells in good health. A steady intake of certain vitamins may also help guard against chronic diseases like heart disease, cataract, macular degeneration and certain cancers. Of the 13 vitamins we require, two deserve special attention in your plant-based diet.

Vitamin B_{12}

This nutrient is critical for making myelin, the protective sheath that covers our nerves. Vitamin B_{12}, called cobalamin, is also necessary for making and repairing DNA, the genetic material found inside every single cell. And it's used to produce red blood cells; without vitamin B_{12} we'd feel tired, listless and weak. Along with other vitamins, B_{12} helps convert carbohydrate, protein and fat in the foods we eat into energy compounds that the body can use.

Vitamin B_{12} is a nutrient of concern for plant-based eaters because it's not present in plants. Natural vitamin B_{12} is found only in animal foods: meat, poultry, fish, eggs and dairy. Bacteria that live in the intestinal tract of animals produce it. But just because the vitamin is not produced in plants, that doesn't mean it's impossible to get B_{12} in a plant-based diet. Synthetic vitamin B_{12}, called cyanocobalamin, is added to some fortified vegetarian foods and you'll also find it in supplements. Here's how much you need every day, regardless of the type of diet you follow.

Recommended Dietary Allowances (RDAs) for Vitamin B_{12}

	Vitamin B_{12} (mcg)
Children, 1 to 3 years	0.5
Children, 4 to 8 years	0.9
Children, 9 to 13 years	1.2
Males and females, 14+ years	2.4
During pregnancy	2.6
While breastfeeding	2.8
Safe upper limit	None

VITAMIN B_{12} IN A PLANT-BASED DIET

You'll find vitamin B_{12} in fortified plant beverages such as soy, rice, almond, oat and hemp milks. Every 1 cup (250 mL) of these fortified beverages supplies 1 microgram of the vitamin. It's also added to ready-to-eat breakfast cereals and some soy products such as veggie burgers and veggie dogs. You need to check the nutrition label to see if vitamin B_{12} is added to these foods. You'll see vitamin B_{12} listed as a percentage of a Daily Value (DV). For example, one Yves Veggie Cuisine Prima Veggie Burger (75 g) contains 40 percent of the DV for vitamin B_{12}. For nutrition-labelling purposes, the daily value for vitamin B_{12} is 2 micrograms. If you do the math, that means that one Yves Prima Veggie Burger has 0.8 micrograms of vitamin B_{12} ($0.4 \times 2 = 0.8$). You can also scan the ingredient list to ensure that synthetic vitamin B_{12} (cyanocobalamin) has been added.

As long as you eat fortified foods or a vitamin B_{12}–containing supplement, you'll be sure to get enough B_{12} in a plant-based diet. It's not hard to do. In fact, I recently analyzed the diet of a vegan client and determined that she consumed 7 micrograms of vitamin B_{12}—more than two days' worth—without taking a supplement! The plant-based menu on page 65, Step 4, provides 3 micrograms of the vitamin.

My advice: Include three servings of vitamin B_{12} in your daily diet. One serving may be any of the following:

- 1/2 cup (125 mL) fortified plant beverage
- 30 grams fortified breakfast cereal
- 42 grams fortified soy product
- 1 tablespoon (15 mL) nutritional yeast (you'll learn more about this yeast in Part 2, *The Plant-Based Power Diet*)

To ensure that you're meeting your daily vitamin B_{12} requirements, you can take a daily multivitamin and mineral supplement that contains 5 to 10 micrograms of B_{12}. Or, you can take a separate vitamin B_{12} supplement of 500 to 1000 micrograms. Vitamin B_{12} supplements are very safe; no adverse effects have been linked to high intakes of vitamin B_{12} from foods or supplements.

VITAMIN B_{12} ABSORPTION FROM FOODS

You may have heard that after age 50 it's necessary to get your vitamin B_{12} from a supplement. That's true for meat eaters who don't eat fortified foods. Here's why: In order for vitamin B_{12} to be absorbed from animal foods, it first must be cleaved from the protein to which it's attached. Hydrochloric acid in your stomach performs this task, making vitamin B_{12} ready for absorption into your bloodstream. As we age, however, we produce less stomach acid and our ability to absorb vitamin B_{12} declines. It's estimated that up to 30 percent of older adults have a condition called atrophic gastritis in which they don't produce nearly enough hydrochloric acid to absorb natural B_{12} from foods. (People who take medication to block the production of stomach acid will also absorb vitamin B_{12} poorly.)

The simple solution is to take a vitamin B_{12}–containing supplement or eat vitamin B_{12}–fortified foods. That's because these products contain synthetic vitamin B_{12}, a form that isn't attached to protein so it's well absorbed by the body. You don't need to worry that your body isn't able to absorb the vitamin on *The Plant-Based Power Diet* since your B_{12} is coming from fortified foods and, if you choose, a multivitamin or B_{12} supplement.

Vitamin D

This fat-soluble vitamin keeps us healthy in many different ways. It helps to maintain strong bones by helping the body absorb calcium from foods. Together with calcium, vitamin D helps protect us from osteoporosis. But there's more to vitamin D than bone health. Our immune system needs vitamin D to fight off invading bacteria and viruses. The nutrient also helps reduce inflammation in the body. Vitamin D is also being studied for its connection to several diseases. Having suboptimal vitamin D blood levels has been linked to diabetes, high blood pressure, heart disease, multiple sclerosis, rheumatoid arthritis and certain cancers, especially colon cancer.

THE SUNSHINE NUTRIENT

If you live in the northern hemisphere like we do in Canada, you're at risk for vitamin D deficiency whether or not you eat a plant-based diet. That's because our main source of the nutrient is sunlight. When exposed to sunlight, UVB rays activate a cholesterol compound in our skin called 7-dehydrocholesterol, which makes its way to the kidneys where it's transformed into active vitamin D. Then, vitamin D goes to work performing all of its important functions throughout the body. In fact, every cell in the body has receptors for vitamin D, indicating that the nutrient has far-reaching health effects in the body.

During the summer, our bodies store vitamin D for the months ahead, presuming that you've had sun exposure. Vitamin D experts suggest that it takes about 5 to 30 minutes of sun exposure between 10 a.m. and 3 p.m. at least twice a week to the face, arms, legs or back—without sunscreen, which blocks vitamin D synthesis—to produce sufficient vitamin D. However, due to concerns about skin cancer it's prudent to apply sunscreen before going outside and to wear protective clothing. This means you may be getting less vitamin D than you think, even on a sunny day.

During our long, dark winters the sun never gets high enough in the sky for its UVB rays to penetrate the atmosphere. So, if you haven't adequately stocked up on vitamin D during the summer, your blood level can drop too low.

IS YOUR VITAMIN D SUFFICIENT?

The best measure of your vitamin D status is your blood level of a 25-hydroxy vitamin D, a simple blood test your doctor can request. A level of 75 nmol/L (nanomoles per litre) or greater is considered sufficient. Below 75 nmol/L is insufficient, and less than 25 nmol/L indicates vitamin D deficiency. Research suggests that a blood level of 25-hydroxy vitamin D between 90 and 100 nmol/L is optimal for health.

Having a blood level of 25-hydroxy vitamin D greater than 100 nmol/L is not necessarily better. Emerging evidence has linked levels over 125 nmol/L with a greater risk of pancreatic and kidney cancers. Blood levels above 250 nmol/L are associated with vitamin D toxicity, which can cause nausea, vomiting, poor appetite, weakness, heart problems and kidney damage.

HOW MUCH VITAMIN D?

So, how much vitamin D do you need every day? The Recommended Dietary Allowance (RDA) for vitamin D is 600 IU (international units) from ages 1 to 70 (infants require 400 IU per day). At age 71, the RDA increases to 800 IU. However, many people may need more vitamin D to ensure a sufficient blood level. Older adults, people with dark-coloured skin, those with limited sun exposure and obese individuals may need 1000 IU per day or more. The safe upper vitamin D limit for adults is 4000 IU per day.

The only way to know if you're getting enough vitamin D is to have your blood tested by your doctor. But keep in mind that your 25-hydroxy vitamin D level can vary from season to season depending on sun exposure.

GETTING VITAMIN D FROM FOOD

You can't rely on diet to give you enough vitamin D since very few foods contain the nutrient naturally. The best sources are fatty fish like salmon and mackerel and fish-liver-oil supplements. Small amounts are also found in cheese and egg yolks. Fortified foods like milk and margarine provide most of the vitamin D in the North American diet. (In the United States, most breakfast cereals are also fortified with vitamin D.) Vitamin D is also added to some brands of orange juice and many fortified plant-based beverages.

You're probably wondering how to get enough vitamin D in a plant-based diet since the main sources are fish, milk and eggs. The bottom line: You need to take a supplement. Even if you drank a few glasses of fortified soy milk each day, you still wouldn't meet vitamin D intake recommendations. (People who eat fish and drink milk also have trouble getting enough vitamin D through their diet and need to supplement.)

VITAMIN D SUPPLEMENTS

Vitamin D comes in two forms: vitamin D_2 (from plants, usually yeast) and vitamin D_3 (from animals, usually fish oil or sheep's wool). Both increase vitamin D levels in the blood, but studies suggest that at very high doses vitamin D_2 is less potent. At a dose of 1000 IU per day, however, both are effective. If you are vegan, you'll want to take a supplement made from vitamin D_2.

I advise my clients to get 1000 IU of vitamin D per day, unless their 25-hydroxy vitamin D level indicates that they need more to maintain a sufficient level. Keep in mind that multivitamins provide vitamin D, usually 400 IU. If you take calcium supplements, check to see if your product also contains vitamin D. Add up vitamin D from all of your supplements and then make up the difference with a separate vitamin D supplement. Vitamin D typically comes in doses of 400 IU and 1000 IU.

MIGHTY MINERALS

As with vitamins, your body can't make minerals on its own so they must come from your diet. These tiny elements are important players in hundreds and hundreds of metabolic reactions in your body. Many enable hormones and enzymes to function, others help maintain fluid balance and some play a critical role in growth and development. All minerals come from the soil, which is how plants accumulate them. By eating plants we, in turn, get plenty of minerals. (Animals get their minerals by eating plants, too.)

The problem is that certain minerals like calcium, iron and zinc are absorbed less well from plant foods than animal foods. Natural compounds in plants called phytates and oxalates bind to minerals, reducing how much your body can absorb and use. The good news: There are a number of ways you can increase mineral absorption from a plant-based diet and get the amount your body needs each day. Of the 22 minerals, I've highlighted three you need to focus on.

Calcium

Calcium is well known for its ability to help maintain strong bones and guard against osteoporosis. But getting enough calcium each day can protect your health in other ways, too. A calcium-rich diet can help prevent—and even lower—high blood pressure, calcium oxalate kidney stones and colorectal cancer. And if you experience premenstrual syndrome, an adequate calcium intake can help ease your symptoms.

You'll find detailed information about calcium in Step 7. In fact, I've devoted that entire step to the topic of calcium. On pages 98–108, you'll find everything you need to know. You'll learn how much calcium you need, what plant-based foods provide the most, how to maximize absorption and tips for safe supplementing.

Iron

Iron is essential for transporting oxygen to the body's tissues. Most of the iron in your body—about two-thirds—is found in hemoglobin, the pigment in red blood cells that shuttles oxygen to all of the cells in your body. Iron also helps enzymes produce energy for cells and supports immune function. As well, the mineral is used to make certain brain chemicals called neurotransmitters that help us concentrate and learn.

Iron deficiency is the most common nutrient deficiency in the world, particularly among premenopausal women, who lose iron each month during menstruation. Iron deficiency usually develops in stages, so it can take months, or even years, before symptoms appear. The main symptoms include fatigue, weakness, loss of appetite, loss of energy, shortness of breath and increased susceptibility to infection. You can feel symptoms even if you are not classified as anemic, which is diagnosed by having a low level of hemoglobin in the blood. A marginal iron deficiency, indicated by a low blood ferritin level, can affect your energy levels as well, although not as severely.

IRON IN PLANT FOODS

When you think of iron, you undoubtedly think of red meat. It's true that red meat is one of the best sources of well-absorbed iron, but a plant-based diet can deliver on iron, too. In fact, plant-based diets actually tend to be higher in iron than those based on animal foods! There are two types of iron in foods: *heme* and *non-heme iron*. Heme iron is present in animal foods and it's the type that can be absorbed and used most efficiently by the body. Plant foods like legumes, nuts, leafy greens and dried fruit supply non-heme iron, a form that's less well absorbed.

Iron-Rich Foods in a Plant-Based Diet

	Iron (mg)
Legumes	
Baked beans in tomato sauce, 1 cup (250 mL)	5.0
Black beans, cooked, 1 cup (250 mL)	3.6
Garbanzo beans, cooked, 1 cup (250 mL)	4.7
Kidney beans, cooked, 1 cup (250 mL)	0.9
Lentils, cooked, 1 cup (250 mL)	6.6
Lima beans, cooked, 1/2 cup (125 mL)	4.2
Navy beans, cooked, 1 cup (250 mL)	2.1
Pinto beans, cooked, 1 cup (250 mL)	0.7
Soybeans, cooked, 1 cup (250 mL)	8.8
Soy burger, 1 patty (70 g)	1.7
Soy nuts, 1/4 cup (50 mL)	1.7
Tempeh, cooked, 3 1/2 ounces (100 g)	2.1
Tofu, firm, 1 cup (250 mL)	4.0
Nuts and seeds	
Almonds, whole, 1/4 cup (50 mL)	1.3
Almond butter, 2 tbsp (25 mL)	1.2
Brazil nuts, 1/4 cup (50 mL)	0.8
Cashews, 1/4 cup (50 mL)	1.7
Mixed nuts, 1/4 cup (50 mL)	1.3
Peanuts, 1/4 cup (50 mL)	0.9
Peanut butter, 2 tbsp (25 mL)	0.7
Pumpkin seeds, 1/4 cup (50 mL)	2.8
Sunflower seeds, shelled, 1/4 cup (50 mL)	0.6
Tahini (sesame seed butter), 2 tbsp (25 mL)	1.6
Walnuts, 1/4 cup (50 mL)	0.7

	Iron (mg)
Breads, grains and cereals	
100% whole wheat bread, 2 slices	1.7
Pita, whole wheat, 6 1/2-inch pocket	2.0
All-Bran, Kellogg's, 1/2 cup (125 mL)	4.7
Shreddies, 3/4 cup (175 mL)	5.4
Bran Flakes, 3/4 cup (175 mL)	3.4
Raisin Bran, 3/4 cup (175 mL)	5.5
Cheerios, 3/4 cup (175 mL)	3.4
Oatmeal, large flake, cooked, 1 cup (250 mL)	1.8
Oatmeal, instant, 1 pouch	4.5
Red River, cooked, 1 cup (250 mL)	1.9
Wheat germ, 2 tbsp (25 mL)	1.3
Barley, cooked, 1 cup (250 mL)	2.2
Brown rice, cooked, 1 cup (250 mL)	0.9
Bulgur, cooked, 1 cup (250 mL)	1.8
Kasha (roasted buckwheat groats), cooked, 1 cup (250 mL)	1.4
Millet, cooked, 1 cup (250 mL)	1.2
Quinoa, cooked, 1 cup (250 mL)	2.2
Whole wheat spaghetti, cooked, 1 cup (250 mL)	1.6
Fruit and vegetables	
Apricots, dried, 1/4 cup (50 mL)	2.0
Dates, dried, 6	0.5
Prunes, dried, 1/4 cup (50 mL)	4.9
Prune juice, 1/2 cup (125 mL)	1.6
Raisins, 1/4 cup (50 mL)	2.0
Strawberries, sliced, 1 cup	0.7
Broccoli, cooked, 1 cup (250 mL)	1.1
Collard greens, cooked, 1 cup (250 mL)	2.3
Kale, cooked, 1 cup (250 mL)	1.2
Spinach, cooked, 1 cup (250 mL)	6.8
Spinach, frozen, cooked, 1 cup (250 mL)	3.9

	Iron (mg)
Spinach, raw, 1 cup (250 mL)	0.9
Potato, Russet, 1 medium, baked in skin	1.9
Sweet potato, 1 medium, baked, no skin	0.8
Tomato juice, 1 cup (250 mL)	1.1

Other	
Blackstrap molasses, 1 tbsp (15 mL)	3.6

Source: USDA Agricultural Research Service. National Agricultural Library. National Nutrient Database for Standard Reference, Release 25. 2012.

I told you earlier that phytates in plant foods bind to iron, reducing its absorption. Other factors in your diet, such as calcium, and tannins in tea, also can inhibit iron absorption. Luckily, there are ways to enhance iron absorption from foods.

Quick Tips to Maximize Iron Absorption from Plants

- Eat some of your foods cooked (e.g., veggies), sprouted (e.g., breads, grains and legumes) and fermented (e.g., tempeh) since these preparation methods release iron from phytates.
- Add a source of vitamin C at every meal. Vitamin C boosts non-heme iron absorption by as much as fourfold. The acidity of the vitamin converts iron in food into a form that's ready for absorption (your stomach acid enhances iron absorption in the same way). Excellent sources of vitamin C include cantaloupe, citrus fruit, mango, strawberries, bell peppers, broccoli, Brussels sprouts, cauliflower, tomato sauce and tomato juice.
- Drink tea between rather than during meals; tea contains tannins, compounds that inhibit iron absorption. Or, add a little milk or lemon to your cup of tea, since both inactivate its iron-binding properties.
- If you take a calcium supplement, don't take it with an iron-rich meal, since these two minerals compete with each other for absorption. If you use calcium citrate supplements, they can be taken between meals. (Refer to page 104 for more on calcium supplements.)

HOW MUCH IRON DO YOU NEED?

Since plant foods contain non-heme iron that's harder for the body to absorb than the heme iron in animal foods, plant-based eaters have higher daily iron requirements to ensure that they get enough. That's why the Recommended Dietary Allowance (RDA) is 1.8 times higher for vegetarians. But keep in mind that this RDA was established based on a low vitamin C intake. *The Plant-Based Power Diet* is high in vitamin C, so you will likely require less than the official RDA. As long as you're eating a variety of plant foods each day, you don't need to take a separate iron supplement. (Keep in mind that a multivitamin and supplement mineral will also provide some of your daily iron.) If you are iron deficient, however, you will need an iron supplement. Speak to your doctor or dietitian about supplementing safely with iron.

Here's how much iron the Institute of Medicine recommends that plant-based eaters get in their daily diets.

Recommended Dietary Allowances (RDAs) for Iron

	Iron (mg)
Children, 1 to 3 years	13
Children, 4 to 8 years	18
Children, 9 to 13 years	14
Boys, 14 to 18 years	20
Girls, 14 to 18 years	27
Males, 19+ years	14
Females, 19 to 50 years	32
Females, 51+ years	14
During pregnancy	48
While breastfeeding	16

Zinc

While you need only a tiny amount of zinc each day, the mineral plays a vital role in many bodily processes. During infancy, childhood and pregnancy, the body needs zinc to grow properly. The mineral is also necessary for a strong immune system, helping us to fight off infection. As well, zinc is used to make DNA in cells and hundreds of body proteins and enzymes. And without zinc, our body wouldn't be able to heal wounds properly.

Like iron, absorption of zinc from plant foods is much lower than from animal foods due to the presence of phytates that keep the mineral from being fully absorbed. Zinc deficiency is rare in North America and there's no evidence that plant-based eaters suffer from such a deficiency. Even so, it's important to include zinc-rich foods in your daily diet and take steps to maximize its absorption.

ZINC IN FOODS

While the best sources of zinc are oysters, meat, poultry and seafood, plant foods such as legumes, nuts and grains provide some zinc, too. Eating fortified breakfast cereals and drinking fortified plant beverages are other ways to add zinc to a plant-based diet.

Zinc-Rich Foods in a Plant-Based Diet

	Zinc (mg)
Legumes	
Baked beans, 1 cup (250 mL)	1.9
Black beans, cooked, 1 cup (250 mL)	1.9
Garbanzo beans, cooked, 1 cup (250 mL)	2.5
Lentils, cooked, 1 cup (250 mL)	2.5
Lima beans, 1/2 cup (125 mL)	1.3
Soybeans, cooked, 1 cup (250 mL)	2.0
Soy beverages, fortified, 1 cup (250 mL)	1.0
Soy burger, commercial, 1 patty (70 g)	0.9
Soy nuts, 1/4 cup (50 mL)	1.4
Tempeh, cooked, 3 1/2 ounces (100 g)	1.6
Tofu, firm, 1 cup (250 mL)	2.1

	Zinc (mg)
Nuts and seeds	
Almonds, 1/4 cup (50 mL)	1.2
Almond butter, 2 tbsp (25 mL)	1.0
Brazil nuts, 1/4 cup (50 mL)	1.4
Cashews, 1/4 cup (50 mL)	1.9
Peanuts, 1/4 cup (50 mL)	1.2
Peanut butter, 2 tbsp (25 mL)	1.0
Pumpkin seeds, 1/4 cup (50 mL)	2.7
Sunflower seeds, shelled, 1/4 cup (50 mL)	1.8
Tahini (sesame seed butter), 2 tbsp (25 mL)	1.4
Walnuts, 1/4 cup (50 mL)	0.8
Breads, cereals and grains	
Bread, 100% whole wheat, 2 slices	1.0
Pita, whole wheat, 6 1/2-inch pocket	1.0
Bran Flakes, 3/4 cup (175 mL)	1.5
Oats, large flake, cooked, 1 cup (250 mL)	1.6
Brown rice, cooked, 1 cup (250 mL)	1.2
Millet, cooked, 1 cup (250 mL)	1.6
Quinoa, cooked, 1 cup (250 mL)	2.0
Wheat germ, 2 tbsp (25 mL)	2.4

Source: USDA Agricultural Research Service. National Agricultural Library. National Nutrient Database for Standard Reference, Release 25. 2012.

HOW MUCH ZINC DO YOU NEED?

Because zinc is poorly absorbed from plant foods, it's thought that people who eat a 100 percent plant-based diet need to eat as much as 50 percent more zinc than recommended amounts. As a result, the recommended daily zinc intake for plant-based eaters is as follows.

Daily Zinc Requirements in a Plant-Based Diet

	Zinc (mg)
Children, 1 to 3 years	4.5
Children, 4 to 8 years	7.5
Children, 9 to 13 years	12.0
Boys, 14 to 18 years	16.5
Girls, 14 to 18 years	13.5
Males, 19+ years	16.5
Females, 19+ years	12.0
During pregnancy	16.5
While breastfeeding	18.0

You don't need to take a zinc supplement to meet your daily needs. In fact, taking too much zinc for a long time can cause low copper levels, lower immunity and reduced levels of HDL (good) cholesterol. A varied diet—along with a multivitamin and mineral supplement—will supply all of the zinc you need. It's also important to optimize zinc absorption from foods. Use the tips on page 119 to help you boost your body's absorption of both zinc and iron.

Quick Tips to Maximize Your Nutrient Intake from a Plant-Based Diet

- To meet vitamin B_{12} requirements, include three servings of vitamin B_{12}–rich foods in your daily diet. One serving is equivalent to 1/2 cup (125 mL) of a fortified plant beverage, 30 grams of a fortified breakfast cereal, 42 grams of a fortified soy product (e.g., soy burger, soy hot dogs, etc.) or 1 tablespoon (15 mL) of nutritional yeast.
- To ensure that you're covered for vitamin B_{12}, take a daily multivitamin that contains 5 to 10 micrograms of the vitamin or take a separate vitamin B_{12} supplement.
- Use a fortified plant beverage to add a good source of calcium to your diet. Follow the tips on page 107, Step 7, to add other calcium-rich plant foods to your diet.

- Take 1000 IU (international units) of vitamin D each day to help achieve a sufficient blood level of the nutrient. Add up vitamin D supplied by other supplements you take, such as a multivitamin or calcium pills, and make up the difference with a vitamin D supplement.
- To boost your iron intake, include a variety of legumes, nuts, grains and fortified cereals in your diet. If you're a premenopausal woman, take a multivitamin and mineral supplement each day to provide additional insurance against iron deficiency.
- Add a variety of zinc-rich foods, outlined on pages 121–122, to your plant-based diet.
- To enhance your body's ability to absorb iron and zinc from plant foods, eat your vegetables cooked more often than raw. Try sprouted grains and legumes, which have a higher content of absorbable minerals.
- Drink tea between rather than with meals to boost iron and zinc absorption.
- If you rely on a calcium supplement to meet daily needs, take it apart from meals to prevent the mineral from reducing iron and zinc absorption. Choose a supplement made from calcium citrate, which is well absorbed when taken on an empty stomach. (Calcium carbonate supplements are best absorbed when taken with a meal or immediately after.)

It's now time to discover a whole new world of plant-based eating! The next step of *The Plant-Based Power Diet* will give you all of the tips and tools you need to follow a whole foods, plant-based diet plan that provides all of the nutrients your body needs. Let's get started!

Step 9

Transition to
The Plant-Based Power Diet

Now that you've made up your mind to shift to a plant-based diet, you're probably wondering how to begin. Moving to a 100 percent plant-based diet may even seem like a daunting task to you. While some people choose to go plant-based overnight, others prefer to ease into it gradually. And that's perfectly fine. Depending on where you're starting from, you may find that your transition from a meat-centred diet is much easier than you would think. And not to worry: You don't have to eat exotic foods you've never heard of, nor do you need to spend hours in the kitchen following complicated recipes to make the transition.

The tips in this chapter will allow you to make the changeover at a pace that's comfortable for you. As you begin your journey toward plant-based eating, make small, realistic dietary changes and then build on them one day and one meal at a time.

EAT MORE OF THE PLANT-BASED
MEALS ALREADY ON YOUR MENU

Start with what you're familiar with. Chances are good you already eat 100 percent plant-based meals, even if infrequently. Popular plant-based meals that my clients enjoy include pasta primavera, vegetable curry, veggie burgers, tofu stir-fry, veggie chili and meal-sized salads with chickpeas. A breakfast of fruit and whole-grain toast spread with nut butter may be a plant-based meal you're already eating. A baked potato topped with steamed or sautéed broccoli is another example of a quick plant-based meal. So is a bowl of lentil or black bean soup served with a green salad.

Take a moment to think about your family's usual meals. Identify plant-based meals you are already eating and then rotate them into your menu more often. Introduce plant-based meals on a regular basis by instituting a "meatless Monday."

SHIFT THE FOCUS OF YOUR PLATE

If meat, poultry and fish make up the balance of your meal, downsize their importance. Three-quarters of your plate should be filled with plant foods like grains, legumes, fruit and vegetables. Aim for all of your meals to be 75 percent plant-based.

To do so, add more plant foods to the mixed meals you're eating. Add fruit to breakfast. Ensure that every lunch and dinner includes grains and plenty of vegetables. Increasing the proportion of plant foods at your meals means you'll be cutting back on your intake of animal foods.

ELIMINATE ANIMAL FOODS YOU DON'T EAT OFTEN

Think about your diet. Is there an animal food—or two—that you eat infrequently? Red meat? Eggs? Milk? This will be the easiest food to drop completely—you won't miss it. For many of my clients—myself included—red meat is the first to go. Naturally, many people lean away from meat after realizing the health problems associated with high meat intake. And as they get older, people often complain that they don't feel as good as they used to after eating meat; it takes longer to digest.

MODIFY YOUR FAVOURITE MEALS

To make your transition easier, modify your favourite meals to make them 100 percent plant-based. Instead of serving chicken tacos, try black bean tacos with all of the fixings. Instead of spaghetti with meat sauce, serve spaghetti with a vegetable-packed marinara sauce. A sauce full of red peppers, onions, carrots and spinach leaves is just as sustaining as one that contains meat and scant vegetables. The next time you make a beef or turkey chili, replace the meat with an extra two cans of beans.

If cheese and tomato sandwiches are regular fare, swap the cheese for extra vegetables like cucumber and sprouts and spread with hummus (chickpea spread). Order your next pizza without cheese and add plenty of vegetables—roasted red pepper, grilled zucchini and eggplant, broccoli and onions make for a delicious veggie pizza.

These are only a few ideas. I am sure you can come up with other meal ideas that can easily be converted to plant-based meals. You'll be eating healthier and feeling just as satisfied, if not more so.

EAT FOUR LEGUME MEALS EACH WEEK

Adding bean meals to your weekly menu is a great place to start making the transition. And it's easy, too. I advise all of my clients—whether or not they're moving to a plant-based diet—to include four legume meals in their weekly menu. Bean and lentil soups, chickpea or three bean salad, bean burritos, dahl, pasta with white kidney beans—the list goes on.

You'll find many recipes in *The Plant-Based Power Diet* that turn out delicious-tasting legume meals. Be sure to make my Whole-Grain Lentil Casserole on page 184—my clients can't get enough of this dish! Chipotle Chili (page 176), Three Bean Garden Chili (page 182) and Moroccan Chickpea Stew (page 179) are other favourites. After you try these recipes you'll wonder why you weren't eating legumes more often!

EXPLORE VEGETARIAN COOKBOOKS

Plant-based cookbooks are proliferating. So much so that there are now vegan cookbooks devoted entirely to slow cooker meals, muffins and even vegan entertaining. It just goes to show that plant-based eating is becoming more mainstream.

Find a vegetarian cookbook you like at your local library or bookstore and begin experimenting with new foods and recipes. Or pick up a magazine devoted to vegetarian cooking at the newsstand. Use the tips and recipes in *The Plant-Based Power Diet* as your starting point, but explore other cookbooks and magazines to build on your growing repertoire of plant-based meals.

SWAP YOUR CONDIMENTS

You can always start by making very small changes, changes you won't even notice but that will reduce your intake of animal foods. Why not substitute some of your condiments for plant-based versions? You may have to shop at a natural foods store or at Whole Foods to find some of these products, but many are available in large grocery stores. If your grocer doesn't have a particular item you want, ask that it be ordered in for you.

Try a vegan mayonnaise such as Nayonaise (by Nasoya) or Vegenaise (by Follow Your Heart). Replace cream cheese on toast with a non-dairy version or use nut butter or tahini instead. If you use commercial creamy salad dressings, look for vegan options (although I encourage you to make your own!). For recipes that call for chicken stock, use vegetable stock instead. You'll find many brands of veggie broth on grocery store shelves. Top your next baked potato with a vegan sour cream (Toffuti makes a good one). If you serve gravy with mashed potatoes, use a mushroom gravy. When buying a commercial brand, read labels to choose a lower-sodium product.

THINK CONVENIENCE

Keep it simple when you're starting out. If cooking plant-based meals from scratch seems a bit overwhelming right now, take advantage of the huge selection of vegetarian convenience foods. Many canned and instant bean soups—black bean, lentil, split pea and minestrone—are entirely plant-based. And there are many brands of meatless and cheeseless tomato-based pasta sauces. Walk down the frozen food aisle at a natural foods store and you'll find vegetarian entrees such as tofu lasagna, pad thai, lentil curry, vegetable pot pie, rice and beans, burritos and cheeseless or soy cheese pizzas.

Once you start looking, you'll be amazed at how many choices there are. While these products are convenient and reduce your cooking time, they do come at a cost. While they don't have the saturated fat and cholesterol that their animal-based counterparts do, they can be high in sodium. Be sure to read labels to choose lower-sodium brands. And keep in mind that your ultimate goal is to move to a whole foods, plant-based diet that minimizes processed foods.

RETHINK YOUR RESTAURANT CHOICES

Continue your transition when dining out. If plant-based options are scarce on the menu, ask that a dish be modified. For instance, order a chicken penne dish without chicken and with extra vegetables. Or build a meal from side dishes such as baked potato, rice, steamed vegetables, corn and green salad.

You'll have plenty of options if you try ethnic cuisine. Instead of a steakhouse, try a restaurant that specializes in Italian, Indian, Thai, Japanese, Chinese, Mexican or Middle Eastern cuisine. You'll find that their menus offer a variety of plant-based meals.

EAT PLANT-BASED SNACKS

Making your snack choices plant-based is another step you can take to shift to a 100 percent plant-based diet. Chances are that you're already eating many plant-based snacks. Snack ideas include fruit and nuts, raw veggies and hummus, whole-grain crackers and almond butter, instant bean soups, soy lattes, soy smoothies and plant-based energy bars such Larabar, Kind Bar, Vega Vibrancy Bar and Genuine Health's Vegan Proteins+ Bar.

TRY MEAT SUBSTITUTES

If you crave something "meaty," there are many different plant-based alternatives available in grocery stores. You can add ground soy or texturized vegetable protein (TVP) to pasta sauces, chili and tacos. (You'll learn more about TVP in Step 10.) If it's a burger you want, you'll find soy burgers in the freezer section as well as in the produce section alongside the tofu. As well, there are vegetarian versions of deli meats, bacon, pepperoni, hot dogs, chicken nuggets and even meatballs.

These meat alternatives add a good source of protein to meals without the fat and cholesterol found in meat. But keep in mind that they also bump up the sodium count of your meal, so I wouldn't make them regular fare.

LOOK BEYOND DAIRY

Plant-based beverages are easy to find in any grocery store thanks to consumer demand. And there are many different types. You can choose a plant beverage made from soy, rice, almond, hemp or oats. Fortified products provide just as much calcium as cow's milk. Keep in mind, however, that only soy beverages are a good source of protein, providing 8 to 9 grams per 1 cup (250 mL) serving. Rice, almond, hemp and oat milks contain only a little protein, usually no more than 2 grams per 1 cup (250 mL).

Plant beverages are a simple substitution for cow's milk. In fact, you may already be using one. Use a milk alternative any time you'd normally use dairy milk: over cold or hot cereals, in smoothies and shakes, in French toast and pancake recipes, in cream-style soups and in coffee and tea. Creamier plant beverages like soy milk can also be used to make creamy pasta sauces and desserts such as puddings and custards.

Each type of plant beverage has its own unique taste and texture. Experiment to find one you like. Buy a fortified brand to ensure that you're getting the same vitamins and minerals in dairy milk, and ideally buy an unflavoured or unsweetened product.

Try non-dairy cheeses, too. There are many brands popping up in supermarkets and natural food stores.

LEARN TO COOK WITHOUT EGGS

There are a number of ways to replace eggs in recipes. You can buy powdered egg-free egg replacers in natural food stores. (Bob's Red Mill and Ener-G Foods both make one.) Mixed with water, they can be used to replace eggs in baked products. Or, you can replace one egg in baking with 1 tablespoon (15 mL) of cornstarch plus 2 table-spoons (25 mL) of water. "Egg whites" made from ground flaxseed are another easy egg substitute. To replace one egg, simply whisk 1 tablespoon (15 mL) of ground flaxseed with 3 tablespoons (45 mL) of water until the mixture has a thick, white consistency. Use in sauces or baked goods. Soft tofu can replace eggs, too. To replace one large egg, use 1/4 cup (50 mL) of soft blended tofu.

Step 10

Stock Your Plant-Based Pantry

Adopting a plant-based diet will undoubtedly involve trying new foods and cooking with ingredients you've never used before. But that doesn't mean that many of the items you cook with now can't be part of your new diet. In fact, your pantry may already be well stocked to prepare plant-based meals. In addition to the produce, whole grains, beans and soy foods discussed in Step 3, there are certain ingredients I recommend keeping on hand so you'll be able to whip up a healthy meal quickly. Most are common, easy-to-find items. A few, however, may require a trip to a natural food store or ethnic food market. I've listed the ingredients below in alphabetical order.

BLACKSTRAP MOLASSES
This dark-coloured, thick liquid is a by-product of processing sugar cane into table sugar. It's a good source of minerals, including iron, calcium, magnesium, potassium, manganese and copper. In fact, 1 tablespoon (15 mL) has 180 milligrams of calcium and 3.6 milligrams of iron! Add it to baked beans for extra flavour and nutrients. Or drizzle it over a bowl of hot cereal.

DRIED FRUIT
Dried apricots, raisins, cranberries, dates, figs and other dried fruit make delicious fibre- and nutrient-rich snacks. I also like to add dried fruit to salads, whole-grain pilafs and stews. My Moroccan Chickpea Stew on page 179 includes dried apricots and raisins.

When buying dried fruit, read the ingredient list to be sure there is no added sugar.

EDAMAME

These green young soybeans are a protein-rich food that adults and kids love. You'll find bags of edamame in your grocery store's freezer case. They're sold shelled or still in their pods. Edamame are already cooked; just thaw them and enjoy. Or steam or boil them and eat them hot. Eat edamame as a snack or add them shelled to salads. Try my recipes for Zesty Edamame (page 211) and Sesame Ginger Edamame (page 208).

There's more to edamame than protein. One-half cup of shelled edamame (about 1 1/8 cups in the pods) delivers 11 grams of protein along with 9 grams of fibre. They're also a good source of vitamins A and C and iron.

HERBS AND SPICES

Keep a variety of dried herbs and spices on hand, especially staples used in ethnic cuisine. Coriander, cumin, turmeric, basil, oregano, rosemary, thyme and paprika are must-haves. Spice blends such as chili powder, Chinese five-spice powder, curry powder and garam masala are also worth having in your spice drawer.

Not only do herbs and spices boost the flavour of foods, but many also add disease-fighting phytochemicals to your meal!

HUMMUS

Made from chickpeas and tahini (sesame seed butter), this dip is a staple for many plant-based eaters. And it's easy to make from scratch if you have a good food processor. You'll find my recipe for Lemon Hummus on page 207. You can also buy hummus—plain and in assorted flavours—in the grocery store. Read the ingredient list to find a brand with as few ingredients as possible. Fewer ingredients usually means fewer synthetic additives. When I don't have homemade hummus on hand, my go-to brand is Sunflower Kitchen.

Use hummus as a dip for vegetables and pita chips, as a spread on whole-grain bread and crackers or as an ingredient in salad dressings.

LEGUMES

Beans and lentils are a prominent part of a plant-based diet. Stock your pantry with a variety of dried and canned beans. You'll need dried green lentils for my Whole-Grain Lentil Casserole recipe on page 184. Dried red and yellow lentils are quick cooking and make a great addition to soups. Refer to page 42 in Step 3 for instructions on how to cook dried legumes.

Keep cans of kidney beans, black beans, soybeans, pinto beans, chickpeas and lentils on hand for making chilis and tacos and adding to salads. They're so convenient—all you need to do is drain and rinse them well before adding to a recipe or meal.

MEAT ANALOGUES

Mock meats like soy ground round and soy burgers as well as countless types of vegetarian deli meats, meatballs, turkey slices and hot dogs are other items you may want to have in your fridge or freezer. They're intended to imitate the texture, appearance and flavour of meat. They're made from non-animal ingredients, mainly soy, so they're void of saturated fat and cholesterol. But because they are processed foods, they can add considerable sodium to your diet. Read labels to choose lower-sodium brands.

MISO

This staple in Japanese and Chinese cooking is a thick paste made from soybeans, sea salt and koji (a starter) and often mixed with rice, barley or another grain. The mixture is then fermented, which results in a product with beneficial probiotic bacteria. Miso varies in colour and taste; in general, the darker the colour, the stronger the taste. You'll find miso in the refrigerator section of your super-market. It's also widely available in Asian grocery stores.

Miso has a tangy, salty flavour that's a wonderful addition to many recipes. You can add it to salad dressings, marinades and, of course, miso soup. Or thin the miso with cooking water and use it as a sauce for roasted or sautéed vegetables. It's also great when added to dipping sauces for spring rolls and raw vegetables.

MUSHROOMS
The earthy, robust flavour and dense texture of mushrooms make them a good alternative to meat. I just love the taste of grilled portobello mushrooms. Serve them in hamburger buns or enjoy them on their own as part of your meal. You'll find my recipe for Grilled Balsamic Portobello Mushrooms on page 197. Brown (cremini) mushrooms add depth to any marinara sauce; I find they have more flavour than white mushrooms. Try sliced oyster and shiitake mushrooms in Asian-inspired stir-fries and soups.

Dried mushrooms such as porcini and morels also add extra flavour to pasta sauces, lasagnas, risottos and soups. And they're much less expensive than buying these mushrooms fresh when they're in season.

NON-DAIRY MILKS
Plant beverages made from soy, rice, almonds, hemp and oats are sold fresh in the dairy case or in shelf-stable aseptic packages on grocery store shelves. Soy beverages are a good source of protein, while most other plant-based beverages are not. Whichever you choose, buy a product that's fortified with vitamins and minerals. To limit refined sugar, choose one that's unflavoured (contains very little added sugar) or unsweetened (contains no added sugar).

Use non-dairy milks the same way you'd use cow's milk—on cereal, in smoothies and in coffee and tea. Use them in cooking and baking, too: Substitute non-dairy milks for cow's milk in soups, casseroles, pancake batters and muffin and quick bread recipes.

NUTS AND SEEDS
A plant-based diet wouldn't be complete without a selection of nuts and seeds. Toasted nuts are delicious when added to salads, stir-fries and sautéed leafy greens. Raw sunflower and pumpkin seeds are also great in a green salad. Chopped pecans and walnuts

are easy additions to cookie and quick bread recipes. Some of my clients even sprinkle ground almonds over a bowl of hot cereal or add them to a soy smoothie. And, of course, nuts and seeds make a great protein-rich snack.

Staples in my pantry include pine nuts, almonds (slivered and whole), walnuts, pecans, sunflower seeds, pumpkin seeds and sesame seeds. Buy nuts and seeds raw or dry roasted and unsalted. Once opened, store packages of nuts in the refrigerator to prevent spoilage.

NUT BUTTERS

Peanut, almond, cashew, macadamia and hazelnut butters add protein, vitamins and minerals to a plant-based diet. Look for natural nut butters that are free of added oils and stabilizers. Once opened, natural nut butters should be stored in the fridge for up to six months. That's because oils in nuts are sensitive to light and heat and will go rancid more quickly at room temperature. Natural nut butters have a tendency to separate, the oil floating to the top of the nut butter. Storing them in the fridge will help prevent this.

Spread nut butter on toast, sliced apple or celery sticks. They also add flavour to smoothies and shakes. Add nut butter to muffin, cookie and granola bar recipes. Make your own peanut sauce to serve with grilled tofu or a peanut salad dressing to drizzle over a tofu salad.

NUTRITIONAL YEAST

This special type of yeast is grown on sugar cane or beet molasses. At the end of the growing process, the yeast is killed so it doesn't have the leavening power of live yeast used to make bread. Nutritional yeast lends a nutty, cheesy flavour to dishes, not to mention plenty of B vitamins, especially vitamin B_{12}. It's sold in natural food stores as flakes, small or large. Red Star is a well-known brand of nutritional yeast.

Sprinkle nutritional yeast flakes over pasta in place of Parmesan cheese. Or top a bowl of popcorn with a few flakes. Nutritional yeast can be added to just about any food for a boost of flavour and B vitamins.

OILS

Healthy unsaturated cooking oils to keep in your pantry include canola oil (a source of the omega-3 fatty acid called alpha-linolenic acid) and extra virgin olive oil (an excellent source of monounsaturated fat). Roasted sesame oil is great to have on hand to add flavour to stir-fries—all you need is a drizzle. I also like to keep a bottle of walnut oil handy to add nutty flavour and omega-3s to a vinaigrette salad dressing. If you like, flaxseed oil can be used as a supplemental source of alpha-linolenic acid; one teaspoon provides more than a day's worth! Store sesame, walnut and flaxseed oils in the fridge to prolong their shelf life.

SEITAN

Often called wheat gluten, seitan is made from wheat flour or vital wheat gluten. It's made by rinsing away the starch from the wheat, leaving behind a high-protein gluten that resembles the look and texture of meat. You can make it at home from scratch or you can buy commercially prepared seitan in the refrigerated section of natural food stores.

Add seitan to casseroles, soups, grain pilafs, stir-fries, curries and pasta sauces. It can also be marinated and grilled on the barbecue.

TAHINI

This creamy paste, similar to peanut butter, is made from ground sesame seeds. It's rich in calcium and is a staple ingredient in Middle Eastern cooking. Tahini is typically sold in glass jars with other nut butters, but you can also find it fresh in the refrigerated section of large grocery stores next to the hummus. Store tahini in the refrigerator.

Tahini is a common ingredient in hummus and baba ghanouj (a popular dip made from eggplant) recipes. It can also be added to vegetarian salad dressing and sauces for vegetables. I also enjoy tahini on whole-grain toast as a change from nut butter. Try my Falafel Wrap with Lemon Tahini Sauce on page 177.

TEMPEH

Tempeh is made from cooked and fermented soybeans and pressed into cakes or blocks that can be sliced or crumbled and added to recipes. Many tempeh products have added grains, spices and flavours. Tempeh is sold in the refrigerated section of natural food stores and large grocery stores.

Like tofu, tempeh is a good source of protein and calcium. But unlike tofu, tempeh has a nutty flavour and chewy texture. If you don't like the mild taste of tofu, you may love the flavour of tempeh. Add cubes of tempeh to a stir-fry or crumble it into soups, tacos, burritos and chilis. To introduce tempeh to your diet, try Tempeh Vegetable Summer Rolls on page 191.

TEXTURIZED VEGETABLE PROTEIN (TVP)

This meat alternative is made from defatted soy flour and sometimes fillers such as wheat or oats. TVP varies in size; it's sold as dried flakes or in medium or large chunks. Because it's a dehydrated product, TVP needs to be reconstituted in hot water or broth for about 10 minutes, or during the cooking process, before eating it. It's very versatile and, like tofu, will take on the flavour of the liquid and spices in which it's cooked.

TVP works well in recipes where you'd use ground meat—pasta sauces, tacos, burritos, casseroles and chilis. Note that TVP made with wheat is not gluten-free.

TOFU

Also known as soybean curd, tofu is a protein powerhouse in a plant-based diet. It can also be a great source of calcium if you choose a tofu made with calcium sulphate (check the ingredient list). Made from soybeans, water and a curdling agent, tofu has mild flavour that takes on the flavour of any dish to which it's added.

Regular tofu is available soft, medium or firm. Use firm or extra-firm tofu in stir-fries, curries or any dish where you want the tofu to retain its shape. Firm tofu is delicious baked or grilled. Try my recipe for Spicy Baked Tofu on page 190. Soft tofu is a good choice for recipes that call for blended tofu like lasagne, smoothies and salad dressings. Silken tofu is made by a slightly different process that produces a creamy, custard-like product. It's best suited for salad dressings, sauces and desserts.

VEGETABLE BROTH
Always have canned or boxed vegetable broth on hand to use in place of chicken or beef broth in recipes. Popular brands include Imagine Organic, Pacific Foods, Campbell's and President's Choice Organics. If you're going to follow the 10 percent–fat *Plant-Based Power Diet*, use vegetable broth in place of oil for sautéing. Be sure to read labels to choose a lower-sodium product.

VINEGARS
I couldn't be without my selection of vinegars to add flavour to foods without extra fat or sodium. I use them to flavour salad dressings, marinades and steamed or sautéed leafy greens. (Try my Balsamic Swiss Chard on page 194!) My collection includes the usuals— balsamic and red wine vinegars—but also champagne vinegar, raspberry vinegar (tastes great splashed over steamed spinach), rice vinegar and seasoned rice vinegar. Use seasoned rice vinegar as a stand-alone fat-free salad dressing—it adds flavour without oil. (Look for a brand of seasoned rice vinegar that is low in sodium, ideally no more than 60 milligrams per tablespoon.)

WHOLE GRAINS
The wide selection of whole grains available today in grocery stores is incredible. And that's good news since whole grains are the backbone of a plant-based diet. Whether it's a bowl of steel-cut oats at breakfast, hummus on sprouted grain bread at lunch or a quinoa pilaf at dinner, whole grains feature prominently in *The Plant-Based Power Diet*.

Keep your pantry stocked with oats (large flake or steel-cut), brown rice, quinoa, whole-grain couscous, hulled barley (pearled barley is refined) and whole wheat pasta. But be adventurous and try whole grains you haven't tasted before—bulgur, farro, millet, rye berries and roasted buckwheat (kasha) are only a few of the whole grains you'll find on grocery store shelves.

PART 2
The Plant-Based Power Diet

The Plant-Based Power Diet
Food Groups and Serving Sizes

The Plant-Based Power Diet is built on five food groups: Legumes and Soy, Grains and Starchy Vegetables, Fruit, Vegetables and Healthy Fats and Oils. Within each food group you'll find whole foods rich in fibre, vitamins, minerals and antioxidants that are virtually free from saturated fat and cholesterol. And, of course, all are naturally low in sodium.

It's important to eat a variety of foods from each of the food groups to meet your daily nutrient requirements. And don't forget about the nutritional superstars in the Vegetable and Fruit food groups that I highlighted on pages 25–40. Include these disease-fighting foods in your diet on a regular basis. Here are the key nutrients that each food group provides:

- **Legumes and Soy:** protein, carbohydrate, fibre, folate, calcium, magnesium, iron, zinc, phytochemicals
- **Grains and Starchy Vegetables:** carbohydrate, fibre, B vitamins, iron
- **Fruit:** carbohydrate, fibre, vitamins A and C, folate, potassium, phytochemicals
- **Vegetables:** fibre, vitamins A and C, folate, calcium, magnesium, potassium, phytochemicals
- **Healthy Fats and Oils:** unsaturated fat, essential fatty acids, vitamin E

The Plant-Based Power Diet meal plans on pages 151–152 indicate how many servings from each food group you should eat each day—how you should combine them at meals to help stabilize your blood sugar and maximize your energy after eating. Below, I have highlighted good sources (✓✓) of calcium in each food group so you can get plenty of this mineral in your daily diet. (A good source has at least 100 milligrams of calcium per serving.) The meal plans on pages 151–152 indicate how many calcium-rich food servings to eat each day.

You will notice that nuts, seeds and nut butters are included in the Legumes and Soy food group as well as in the Healthy Fats and Oils food group. That's because when they're eaten in very small portions—six almonds, for example—they can be counted as one Healthy Fats and Oils serving. But if you are eating nuts in a 1/4 cup (50 mL) serving, they provide similar calories—and in some cases protein—to the indicated serving size of beans and soy foods. In this case, they can be counted toward Legumes and Soy servings, not Healthy Fats and Oils.

The portion size for one serving is listed beside each food. Please note that serving sizes are measured *after* cooking, not before.

Legumes and Soy

	1 serving	Calcium-rich
Black beans	3/4 cup (175 mL)	
Black-eyed peas	3/4 cup (175 mL)	✓✓
Chickpeas	3/4 cup (175 mL)	
Kidney beans	3/4 cup (175 mL)	
Lentils	3/4 cup (175 mL)	
Navy beans	3/4 cup (175 mL)	✓✓
Pinto beans	3/4 cup (175 mL)	
Split peas	3/4 cup (175 mL)	
Soybeans, mature	3/4 cup (175 mL)	✓✓
Soybeans, green (edamame)	3/4 cup (175 mL)	✓✓
Soy beverages, fortified, unflavoured	1 cup (250 mL)	✓✓
Soy burger	1 (75 g)	✓✓
Soy ground round	3/4 cup (175 mL)	✓✓
Soy dog	2 small (46 g) or 1 large (75 g)	

	1 serving	Calcium-rich
Soy nuts, roasted	1/4 cup (50 mL)	
Tempeh, cooked	3/4 cup (175 mL)	✓✓
Tofu, firm	3/4 cup (175 mL)	✓✓
Tofu, soft	3/4 cup (175 mL)	✓✓
Texturized vegetable protein (TVP), rehydrated	3/4 cup (175 mL)	
Almonds	1/4 cup (50 mL)	✓✓
Almond butter	2 tbsp (25 mL)	✓✓
Nuts, seeds (whole or chopped)	1/4 cup (50 mL)	
Nut and seed butters	2 tbsp (25 mL)	
Tahini	2 tbsp (25 mL)	✓✓

Grains and Starchy Vegetables

	1 serving
Breads (a whole grain must be the first ingredient)	
Bread	1 slice (30 g)
Bagel, small	1/2 (30 g)
Bagel, regular size	1/4 (30 g)
Bun (e.g., kaiser roll, hamburger roll)	1/2
English muffin	1/2
Pita pocket, 6-inch	1/2 (30 g)
Tortilla, soft, 7-inch	1
Tortilla, soft, 10-inch	1/2

Cereals (a whole grain must be the first ingredient)	
Cold cereal, dry flake (e.g., Bran Flakes, Cheerios, Shreddies, Spoon Size Shredded Wheat)	3/4 cup (175 mL)
Cold cereal, denser flake (e.g., Kashi Go Lean, Nature's Path Flax Plus, Nature's Path Optimum)	1/2 cup (125 mL)

	1 serving
Cold cereal, 100% bran	1/2 cup (125 mL)
Cold cereal, Kellogg's All-Bran Buds with psyllium	1/3 cup (75 mL)
Cold cereal, granola	1/4 cup (50 mL)
Cold cereal, shredded wheat	1 biscuit
Oats, dry	1/4 cup (50 mL)
Oatmeal, cooked	1/2 cup (125 mL)
Oatmeal, instant, unflavoured	1/2 pouch

Crackers

Soda crackers, whole wheat	7
Finn Crisp crackers	3 slices
Rice cakes, brown	2
Rice crackers, brown, small	10
Ryvita crispbread	3 slices
Wasa crackers	1.5 slices

Grains and starchy vegetables

Barley, bulgur, couscous, farro, millet, quinoa, rice	1/3 cup (75 mL)
Corn	1/2 cup or 1/2 cob
Pasta, whole wheat, cooked	1/2 cup (125 mL)
Popcorn, air popped or low-fat microwave	3 cups (750 mL)
Potato, new or yellow flesh	1/2 medium or 1/2 cup (125 mL)
Potato, sweet	1/2 medium or 1/2 cup (125 mL)
Soup, broth-based with potato, grain or pasta	1 cup (250 mL)

Fruit

	1 serving	Calcium-rich
Berries, fresh (blackberries, blueberries, raspberries)	1 cup (250 mL)	
Berries, fresh (cranberries, strawberries)	1 1/2 cups (375 mL)	
Grapes	1 cup (250 mL) or 30 grapes	
Fruit, fresh (apple, pear, kiwifruit, orange, peach, nectarine)	1 medium	
Fruit, fresh (banana, grapefruit)	1 small	
Fruit, fresh (mango, papaya)	1/2 medium	
Fruit, fresh, small (apricots, plums, prunes)	4	
Fruit, fresh, small (figs)	2 small	
Fruit, canned, packed in water	1 cup (250 mL)	
Fruit, dried (apricots)	7 halves	
Fruit, dried (dates, figs)	3	
Fruit, dried (raisins, cranberries)	2 tbsp (25 mL)	
Melon (cantaloupe, honeydew)	1/2 small or 1 cup (250 mL) cubes	
Melon (watermelon, diced)	1 1/2 cups (375 mL)	
Pineapple, fresh or canned in water or juice	3/4 cup (175 mL)	
100% fruit juice (unsweetened)	1/2 cup (125 mL)	
100% fruit juice, calcium fortified	1/2 cup (125 mL)	✓✓

Vegetables

1 serving = 1/2 cup (125 mL) cooked or raw or 1 cup (250 mL) salad greens or 1/2 cup (125 mL) 100% vegetable juice

To maximize your phytochemical intake, choose at least three different-coloured vegetables each day.

✓ Indicates calcium-rich vegetables in 1/2 cup (125 mL) serving size

✓✓ Indicates calcium-rich vegetables in 1 cup (250 mL) serving size

Green	Yellow/Orange	Red
Artichokes	Butternut squash	Beets
Arugula	Carrots	Radicchio
Asparagus	Pumpkin	Radishes
Beet greens ✓	Rutabaga	Red onions
Bok choy ✓	Winter squash	Red peppers
Broccoflower	Yellow peppers	Tomatoes
Broccoli ✓	Yellow summer squash	Tomato juice
Brussels sprouts	Yellow tomatoes	
Celery		
Chinese cabbage		
Collard greens ✓✓		
Cucumbers	**White**	**Blue/Purple**
Endive	Cauliflower	Eggplant
Green beans	Jicama	Purple cabbage
Green cabbage	Cauliflower	Eggplant
Green leaf lettuce	Kohlrabi	Purple carrots
Kale ✓	Mushrooms	Purple endive
Okra ✓	Onions	Purple peppers
Peas	Parsnips	
Rapini ✓✓	Turnips	
Romaine lettuce		
Snow peas		
Spinach ✓✓		
Swiss chard		
Watercress		
Zucchini		

Healthy Fats and Oils

	1 serving
Spreads and dips	
Hummus	2 tbsp (25 mL)
Margarine (non-hydrogenated)	1 tsp (5 mL)
Margarine, light	2 tsp (10 mL)
Pesto sauce (cheeseless)	1 1/2 tsp (7 mL)
Dressings and oils	
Mayonnaise (plant-based; e.g., Nayonaise, Vegenaise)	1 tsp (5 mL)
Salad dressing, vinaigrette	2 tsp (10 mL)
Salad dressing, fat reduced	4 tsp (20 mL)
Vegetable oil (e.g., olive, canola, flaxseed, walnut)	1 tsp (5 mL)
Nuts, seeds and nut butters	
Almonds, whole	6
Brazil nuts	2
Cashews	5
Peanuts	8
Pecan halves	5
Walnut halves	4
Nut and seed butters, tahini	1 1/2 tsp (7 mL)
Seeds	1 tbsp (15 mL)
Other whole, healthy fats	
Avocado	1/8 of one whole
Olives	6 medium

The Plant-Based Power Diet Meal Plans

Now that you've learned about *The Plant-Based Power Diet* food groups and serving sizes, it's time to translate that information into a diet that's right for you. Below are four different meal plans, each one corresponding to a different calorie level. Which meal plan you choose will depend on your gender (men need more calories than women), your current weight (heavier bodies require more calories) and your activity level. If you are very active, you will generally need to eat more calories to fuel your exercise routine. The meal plans below will help you eat a nutrient-packed plant-based diet.

The Plant-Based Power Diet Meal Plans

Food group	Number of servings per day			
	1400 calories	1600 calories	1900 calories	2200 calories
Legumes and Soy	3	3	4	4
Grains and Starchy Vegetables	5	6	7	9
Fruit	3	4	3	4
Vegetables	5 or more	5 or more	5 or more	5 or more
Healthy Fats and Oils	3	4	6	6
Calcium-rich servings	8	8	8	8

WHICH CALORIE LEVEL IS RIGHT FOR YOU?

Ultimately, the meal plan you choose comes down to your activity level, your height, your gender and whether you'd like to maintain your weight or lose or gain a few pounds. Use the following guidelines to decide which meal plan is right for you.

- In general, most females who wish to maintain their weight can choose between 1600 and 1900 calories. Very active females should choose 1900 calories (you exercise for one hour on most days of the week).
- Females who wish to lose excess weight should choose the 1400- or 1600-calorie meal plan.
- Most males should choose the 2200-calorie meal plan. Note, however, that if you are physically active, you may need to increase the number of servings from food groups to get adequate calories.
- Males who wish to lose excess weight can choose between 1900 and 2200 calories. Very active men should select the 2200-calorie meal plan for healthy weight loss.

MEETING NUTRIENT NEEDS ON *THE PLANT-BASED POWER DIET*

Regardless of the calorie level you choose, the following are principal components of your *Plant-Based Power Diet* meal plan.

- **Variety:** Eat a wide variety of foods from each food group to help ensure that you are meeting your daily requirements for essential nutrients.
- **Calcium-rich food choices (✓✓):** Include eight servings each day. Older adults who require 1200 milligrams of calcium each day may benefit by taking a 300-milligram calcium citrate supplement.
- **Vitamin B_{12}:** Include three servings of vitamin B_{12}–rich foods in your daily diet, or take a multivitamin supplement that contains 5 to 10 micrograms of the vitamin. (Refer to page 111, Step 8, for sources of vitamin B_{12}.)
- **Vitamin D:** Get 600 to 1000 international units (IU) of vitamin D_3 each day from a supplement. Some people may need to take more vitamin D to maintain a sufficient blood level. (Refer to

pages 114-115, Step 8, for more information about vitamin D supplementation.)

- **Omega-3 fats:** Take 200 to 400 milligrams of plant-based DHA (docosahexaenoic acid) from algae each day.
- **Multivitamin and mineral supplement:** Menstruating women and women following the 1400-calorie meal plan for weight loss should take a daily multivitamin and mineral supplement to ensure that iron needs are met.
- **Iodine:** If you do not use iodized salt, get 75 to 150 micrograms of iodine per day from a supplement. Note that sea salt is not fortified with iodine.

USING *THE PLANT-BASED POWER DIET* MEAL PLANS

Each meal plan is designed to help you eat a well-balanced, nutrient-rich plant-based diet that includes foods from all five food groups. The meal plans will help you meet your daily requirements for protein and vitamins and minerals, especially calcium and iron. And, of course, each meal plan delivers plenty of fibre and protective phytochemicals. Once you've chosen which meal plan you will follow, you need to map out your daily food servings over the course of the day to keep you feeling satisfied and energetic.

In each example below I have divided the recommended servings of plant-based food groups among meals and snacks. But keep in mind that these are only suggestions. Feel free to balance out your food group servings in a way that suits you. (You will notice, however, that I have included at least one serving of Legumes and Soy at each meal to deliver a good source of plant-based protein.)

1400 Calories

	Breakfast	Lunch	Dinner	Snack(s)
Legumes and Soy	1	1	1	
Grains and Starchy Vegetables	1	2	2	
Fruit	1			2
Vegetables		2+	2+	1
Healthy Fats and Oils		1	1	1
Calcium-rich servings: 8 per day				

1600 Calories

	Breakfast	Lunch	Dinner	Snack(s)
Legumes and Soy	1	1	1	
Grains and Starchy Vegetables	2	2	2	
Fruit	1	1		2
Vegetables		2+	2+	1
Healthy Fats and Oils	1	1	1	1
Calcium-rich servings: 8 per day				

1900 Calories

	Breakfast	Lunch	Dinner	Snack(s)
Legumes and Soy	1	1	2	
Grains and Starchy Vegetables	2	3	2	
Fruit	1	1		1
Vegetables		2+	2+	1
Healthy Fats and Oils	2	2	1	1
Calcium-rich servings: 8 per day				

2200 calories

	Breakfast	Lunch	Dinner	Snack(s)
Legumes and Soy	1	1	2	
Grains and Starchy Vegetables	3	3	2	1
Fruit	1	1	1	1
Vegetables		2+	2+	1
Healthy Fats and Oils	2	2	1	1
Calcium-rich servings: 8 per day				

MOVING FOOD SERVINGS FROM ONE MEAL TO ANOTHER

As I mentioned earlier, your *Plant-Based Power Diet* meal plan is intended to serve only as a guideline to help you balance out your food over the course of a day. The way I have mapped out food servings at meals is designed to help you feel satisfied after meals and to keep your blood sugar levels stable for longer after eating. Your meal plan should be flexible, so you may make the following changes, if you wish:

- You may move one Grains and Starchy Vegetables serving from one meal to another.
- On the 1900- and 2200-calorie meal plans, you may move one Legumes and Soy serving from dinner to lunch or breakfast.
- You may move your servings of Healthy Fats and Oils from one meal to another or from one meal to a snack. For example, if you'd like to have almond butter on whole-grain toast at breakfast, feel free to use one Healthy Fats and Oils serving from lunch or dinner.
- If you prefer to eat a low-fat plant-based diet and limit your intake of Healthy Fats and Oils, make up the missing calories by increasing the number of servings from another food group. In general, two Healthy Fats and Oils servings (90 calories) is equivalent to one Grains and Starchy Vegetables serving, one Fruit serving, or 1/2 cup (125 mL) beans. (Refer to pages 92–94, Step 6, for more information about low-fat, plant-based diets.)
- Feel free to substitute one Grains and Starchy Vegetables serving for one Fruit serving and vice versa.
- You may add more vegetables to any meal you like. Vegetables are unlimited. Each meal plan includes a minimum of five daily servings.

The Plant-Based Power Diet
7-Day Menu Plan

The menu that follows is based on 1900 calories per day. It's designed for most active women and for many men who are relatively inactive or trying to lose weight. If you need to eat fewer—or more—calories each day, simply adjust the plan according to the number of food group servings outlined in *The Plant-Based Power Diet* meal plans on pages 151–152.

Day 1

BREAKFAST

1 cup (250 mL) cooked steel-cut oats
1 tablespoon (15 mL) ground flaxseed
1/4 cup (50 mL) chopped walnuts
1 cup (250 mL) unflavoured, fortified soy beverage
1 cup (250 mL) mixed berries
Coffee, tea or herbal tea

LUNCH

Soy burger in 1 whole wheat pita pocket with 1 tablespoon
(15 mL) hummus; add sliced tomato, cucumber and spinach
Side green salad with 2 teaspoons (10 mL) vinaigrette dressing
1 medium-sized orange
Water

DINNER

1 1/2 cups (375 mL) Chickpea Curry (page 175)
1 cup (250 mL) cooked brown basmati rice
1 cup (250 mL) steamed spinach
Water

SNACKS

1 medium apple, sliced with 1 1/2 tablespoons (22 mL) almond
butter
1 cup (250 mL) raw broccoli florets
Water

Nutrition: 1920 cal, 76 g pro, 67 g total fat (30% cal), 9 g saturated
fat, 277 g carb, 52 g fibre, 10 mg chol, 1349 mg sodium. Plus 6 mcg
vitamin B_{12}, 900 mg calcium, 22.6 mg iron, 15.3 mg zinc

Day 2

BREAKFAST

2 slices whole-grain toast with 2 tablespoons (25 mL) tahini

Soy Smoothie

1 cup (250 mL) unflavoured, fortified soy beverage plus 1/2 banana
plus 1/2 cup (125 mL) frozen strawberries

Coffee, tea or herbal tea

LUNCH

1 1/2 cups (375 mL) Chickpea Curry (leftovers from Day 1
dinner)

1 whole wheat pita

Spinach Salad

2 cups (500 mL) baby spinach, sliced mushrooms, 1/2 cup (125 mL)
sliced strawberries with 4 teaspoons (20 mL) raspberry vinaigrette
dressing

1 pear

Water

DINNER

Grilled Tofu with Sautéed Greens (page 187)

1 cup (250 mL) cooked quinoa

Water

SNACKS

4 dried apricots plus 6 almonds

10 baby carrots

Water

Nutrition: 1931 cal, 84 g pro, 72 g total fat (33% cal), 11 g saturated
fat, 262 g carb, 40 g fibre, 10 mg chol, 1585 mg sodium. Plus 3 mcg
vitamin B$_{12}$, 1197 mg calcium, 47.8 mg iron, 12.4 mg zinc

Day 3

BREAKFAST

1 cup (250 mL) whole-grain cold cereal*

1 sliced banana

1 cup (250 mL) unflavoured, fortified soy beverage

1 slice of whole-grain toast with 1 1/2 teaspoons (7 mL) of nut butter

Coffee, tea or herbal tea

Choose a cereal with at least 5 grams of fibre and no more than 6 grams of sugar per serving.

LUNCH

2 cups (500 mL) black bean soup (homemade or vegetarian store-bought brand*)

2 whole-grain rye crackers (approx. 100 cal; e.g., 2 Wasa crisps)

Green salad with 4 teaspoons (20 mL) vinaigrette dressing

1 medium apple

Water

Choose a store-bought soup with no more than 500 milligrams of sodium per serving.

DINNER

2 cups (500 mL) Whole-Grain Lentil Casserole (page 184)

1 cup (250 mL) sautéed kale (use 2 teaspoons/10 mL canola oil)

1/2 cup (125 mL) steamed carrots

1 cup (250 mL) unflavoured, fortified soy beverage

Water

SNACKS

1/4 cup (50 mL) Black Bean Hummus (page 205)

1 cup (250 mL) raw vegetable sticks

1/4 cup (50 mL) raisins

Water

Nutrition: 1904 cal, 83 g pro, 60 g total fat (28% cal), 8 g saturated fat, 288 g carb, 58 g fibre, 15 mg chol, 1766 mg sodium. Plus 6.2 mcg vitamin B_{12}, 1076 mg calcium, 13 mg iron, 7.4 mg zinc

Day 4

BREAKFAST
Breakfast Burrito
Scramble 3/4 cup (175 mL) soft tofu, chopped green onion and chopped red pepper in non-stick pan. Place in a 10-inch whole wheat tortilla, top with salsa, then wrap and enjoy.
1 cup (250 mL) mixed berries
1/2 cup (125 mL) calcium-fortified orange juice
Coffee, tea or herbal tea

LUNCH
1 1/2 cups (375 mL) Whole-Grain Lentil Casserole (leftovers from Day 3 dinner)
1 cup (250 mL) broccoli florets with 1/4 cup (50 mL) hummus for dip
1 apple
Water

DINNER
Whole-Grain Chickpea Vegetable Toss
Toss together 1 cup (250 mL) cooked grain of your choice (e.g., quinoa, millet, farro, brown rice), 1 cup (250 mL) chickpeas and 1 1/2 cups (375 mL) sautéed vegetables (sauté chopped fresh ginger and garlic in canola oil; add kale, red pepper, sliced carrots and sauté until tender-crisp).
Water

SNACKS
Soy Smoothie
1 cup (250 mL) unflavoured, fortified soy beverage plus 1 small banana plus 1 tablespoon (15 mL) peanut butter

Nutrition: 1885 cal, 80 g pro, 48 g total fat (23% cal), 7 g saturated fat, 291 g carb, 71 g fibre, 11 mg chol, 1644 mg sodium. Plus 3.1 mcg vitamin B_{12}, 1212 mg calcium, 17.8 mg iron, 9.8 mg zinc

Day 5

BREAKFAST

1 toasted whole wheat English muffin topped with 2 tablespoons (25 mL) almond butter and 1 banana, sliced
1 cup (250 mL) fortified vanilla soy beverage
Coffee, tea or herbal tea

LUNCH

Entrée Salad with Edamame
2 to 3 cups (500 to 750 mL) salad greens/cabbage, chopped raw vegetables of your choice, 3/4 cup (175 mL) shelled edamame with 4 teaspoons (20 mL) Asian-style ginger or vinaigrette dressing
1 cup (250 mL) mixed berries
Water

DINNER

1 1/2 cups (375 mL) Chipotle Chili (page 176)
Serve over 1 cup (250 mL) steamed brown rice
Side green salad with 4 teaspoons (20 mL) vinaigrette dressing
Water

SNACKS

4 whole-grain crackers (e.g., Ryvita, Finn Crisp) with 2 tablespoons (25 mL) tahini
Red pepper sticks
Water

Nutrition: 1920 cal, 71 g pro, 71 g total fat (32% cal), 9 g saturated fat, 275 g carb, 54 g fibre, 0 mg chol, 1425 mg sodium. Plus 1 mcg vitamin B$_{12}$, 1032 mg calcium, 17.6 mg iron, 10.3 mg zinc

Day 6

BREAKFAST

1 cup (250 mL) cooked oatmeal (cook in unflavoured, fortified soy beverage)
Top with 1 tablespoon (15 mL) chia seeds, 2 tablespoons (25 mL) raisins and a dash of cinnamon
Coffee, tea or herbal tea

LUNCH

1-1/2 cups (375 mL) Chipotle Chili (leftovers from Day 5 dinner)
2 small (6- or 7-inch) corn or whole wheat flour tortillas
Green side salad with 4 teaspoons (20 mL) vinaigrette dressing
1 fruit serving of your choice
Water

DINNER

1/2 block firm tofu, grilled or stir-fried
1 to 2 cups (250 to 500 mL) Balsamic Swiss Chard (page 194)
1 cup (250 mL) brown rice or other cooked whole grain
Water

SNACKS

1/4 cup (50 mL) almonds plus 4 figs or dates
Water

Nutrition: 1893 cal, 71 g pro, 62 g total fat (29% cal), 7 g saturated fat, 284 g carb, 73 g fibre, 0 mg chol, 1646 mg sodium. Plus 3 mcg vitamin B$_{12}$, 1126 mg calcium, 16.8 mg iron, 10.8 mg zinc

Day 7

BREAKFAST

High-Fibre Soy Smoothie

Purée in blender 1 cup (250 mL) unflavoured fortified soy beverage, 1/2 banana, 1 cup (250 mL) strawberries, 1/2 cup (125 mL) Kellogg's All-Bran Original and ice cubes

2 slices sprouted whole-grain bread toasted with 2 tablespoons (25 mL) nut butter

Coffee, tea or herbal tea

LUNCH

3/4 cup (175 mL) mixed bean salad (e.g., Easy Lentil Salad, page 167) in vinaigrette dressing; serve over a bed of baby romaine or baby spinach

1 whole wheat pita

1 fruit serving of your choice

Water

DINNER

1 veggie burger patty, grilled

1 Quinoa Stuffed Red Bell Pepper (page 193)

1 cup (250 mL) sautéed spinach or collard greens

2 cups (500 mL) mixed berries or fruit

Water

SNACKS

Zesty Edamame (page 211)

1 apple

Water

Nutrition: 1883 cal, 87 g pro, 59 g total fat (28% cal), 8 g saturated fat, 299 g carb, 67 g fibre, 15 mg chol, 1900 mg sodium. Plus 5.4 mcg vitamin B_{12}, 1100 mg calcium, 26 mg iron, 15.4 mg zinc

PART 3
The Plant-Based Power Diet Recipes

Salads

Barley Salad with Lemon, Capers and Black Olives   166
Easy Lentil Salad   167
Kasha, Walnut and Apple Salad with Fresh Mint   168
Mango Cashew Salad   169
Quinoa Tabbouleh   170
Red Grape, Arugula and Toasted Walnut Salad   171
Roasted Beet Salad   172
Sesame Coleslaw   173
Spinach Salad with Strawberries, Pine Nuts and
    Champagne Vinaigrette   174

Mains

Chickpea Curry   175
Chipotle Chili   176
Falafel Wrap with Lemon Tahini Sauce   177
Moroccan Chickpea Stew   179
Mushroom Lentil Patties   180
Three Bean Garden Chili   182
Whole-Grain Lentil Casserole   184
Balsamic Glazed Mushroom and Soy Burgers   185
Grilled Tofu with Sautéed Greens   187
Sesame Crusted Tofu   189
Spicy Baked Tofu   190
Tempeh Vegetable Summer Rolls   191
Quinoa Stuffed Red Bell Peppers   193

Vegetable Sides

Balsamic Swiss Chard   194
Broccoli with Sesame Dressing   195
Garlic Roasted Cauliflower   196
Grilled Balsamic Portobello Mushrooms   197
Maple Dijon Carrots   198
Lemon Swiss Chard   199
Oven Roasted Brussels Sprouts   200
Roasted Gingered Squash   201
Simple Sautéed Spinach with Lemon   202
Spicy Sautéed Kale   203
Spinach with Spicy Peanut Sauce   204

Snacks

Black Bean Hummus   205
Kale Chips with Sea Salt   206
Lemon Hummus   207
Sesame Ginger Edamame   208
Spicy Candied Walnuts   209
Tamari Roasted Almonds   210
Zesty Edamame   211

Desserts

Apple Raspberry Crisp with Maple Oat Topping   212
Chocolate Fruit Fondue   213
Cinnamon Pecan Baked Apples   214
Fresh Berries with Chocolate and Toasted Coconut   215
Tropical Fruit Salad with Lemon Maple Glaze   216

Salads

Barley Salad with Lemon, Capers and Black Olives

If you don't have a bottle of wine open, you can easily substitute the same amount of orange juice for a vitamin C boost.

Serves 6

2 1/2 cups (625 mL) water

1/2 cup (125 mL) dry white wine

1 cup (250 mL) pearl barley

2 tbsp (25 mL) extra virgin olive oil

2 tbsp (25 mL) white wine vinegar

1 tbsp (15 mL) freshly squeezed lemon juice

1 tsp (5 mL) Dijon mustard

1/2 tsp (2 mL) coarse sea salt, or to taste

2 carrots, shredded

1/4 cup (50 mL) sliced pitted black olives

2 tbsp (25 mL) capers

2 green onions, finely sliced

In a medium saucepan, bring water and wine to a boil. Add barley; cover and simmer for 1 hour or until barley is tender. Remove from heat, drain any excess liquid and set aside to cool.

In a small bowl, whisk together olive oil, vinegar, lemon juice, mustard and salt.

Combine barley with carrots, olives, capers and green onion. Drizzle with the vinaigrette, tossing to combine. Cover and refrigerate for 2 hours before serving.

Serve cold or at room temperature.

Per 3/4 cup (175 mL) serving: 192 cal, 4 g pro, 6 g total fat (1 g saturated fat), 30 g carb, 4 g fibre, 0 mg chol, 444 mg sodium

Easy Lentil Salad

This is an easy salad to make, and it's loaded with flavour. It tastes best when made a day or two in advance, so make it on the weekend and pack the leftovers in your lunch during the week for a fibre-rich midday meal.

Serves 4

1/3 cup (75 mL) red wine vinegar

2 tbsp (25 mL) olive oil

2 tsp (10 mL) Dijon mustard

1/2 tsp (2 mL) coarse sea salt

2 cans (19 oz/540 mL each) lentils, drained and rinsed well

1 1/2 cups (375 mL) chopped red bell pepper

1 1/2 cups (375 mL) diced cucumber

1/4 cup (50 mL) finely sliced green onion

In a small bowl, whisk together vinegar, olive oil, mustard and salt.

In a large serving bowl, combine lentils, bell pepper, cucumber and green onion.

Drizzle with dressing and stir to combine.

Cover and refrigerate for at least 2 hours before serving. Serve cold.

Per 1 1/2 cup (375 mL) serving: 306 cal, 18 g pro, 8 g total fat (1 g saturated fat), 43 g carb, 10 g fibre, 0 mg chol, 335 mg sodium

Kasha, Walnut and Apple Salad with Fresh Mint

This flavourful and colourful whole-grain salad is as nice to look at as it is to eat. Ideally, make this salad a day or two in advance of serving to allow the flavours to blend. If you don't have seasoned rice vinegar, apple cider vinegar makes for a tasty alternative.

Serves 6

2 cups (500 mL) water

1 cup (250 mL) kasha

1 apple, diced

2 cups (500 mL) shredded carrot

1/4 cup (50 mL) dried cranberries

1/4 cup (50 mL) walnuts, chopped

1/4 cup (50 mL) finely chopped fresh mint

2 green onions, chopped

2 tbsp (25 mL) seasoned rice vinegar

2 tbsp (25 mL) freshly squeezed lemon juice

1 tbsp (15 mL) Dijon mustard

1 tbsp (15 mL) extra virgin olive oil

1 tsp (5 mL) agave nectar (syrup)

In a large saucepan, heat water to a boil. Add kasha; cover and simmer for 10 to 12 minutes or until most of the liquid has been absorbed. Rinse kasha with cold water and set aside to cool.

Meanwhile, in a large bowl, combine apple, carrot, cranberries, walnuts, mint and green onion.

In a small bowl, whisk together rice vinegar, lemon juice, mustard, olive oil and agave nectar.

Toss kasha with the apple mixture. Drizzle with dressing. Cover and refrigerate until ready to serve.

Per 3/4 cup (175 mL) serving: 190 cal, 5 g pro, 6 g total fat (1 g saturated fat), 32 g carb, 4 g fibre, 0 mg chol, 39 mg sodium

Mango Cashew Salad

This refreshing salad bursting with beta-carotene requires no oil at all!
Be sure to use mangos that are slightly firm so they hold their shape
when you mix the salad.

Serves 4

2 mangos, peeled and cubed

1/2 cup (125 mL) thinly sliced red onion

1/4 cup (50 mL) thinly sliced red bell pepper

16 cashews

1/2 cup (125 mL) chopped cilantro

2 tbsp (25 mL) freshly squeezed lime juice

1/8 tsp (0.5 mL) red pepper flakes, or to taste

In a large bowl, toss together mango, red onion, bell pepper, cashews
and cilantro.

Add lime juice and pepper flakes; toss to coat.

Per 3/4 cup (175 mL) serving: 166 cal, 3 g pro, 7 g total fat
(1 g saturated fat), 26 g carb, 3 g fibre, 0 mg chol, 6 mg sodium

Quinoa Tabbouleh

Tabbouleh is a Middle Eastern salad traditionally made with bulgur, a cracked wheat. I've changed things up and substituted quinoa, a whole grain that's high in protein.

Serves 6

4 cups (1 L) cooked quinoa

1 1/2 cups (375 mL) diced cucumber

1 cup (250 mL) finely chopped parsley

1/4 cup (50 mL) chopped mint

1 cup (250 mL) chopped tomato

2 green onions, chopped

1/4 cup (50 mL) freshly squeezed lemon juice

1 tbsp (15 mL) extra virgin olive oil

3 cloves garlic, crushed

1/2 tsp (2 mL) coarse sea salt, or to taste

In a large bowl, toss together quinoa, cucumber, parsley, mint, tomato, green onion, lemon juice, olive oil, garlic and salt.

Cover and refrigerate for at least 2 hours before serving.

Per 1 cup (250 mL) serving: 191 cal, 6 g pro, 5 g total fat (0 g saturated fat), 32 g carb, 5 g fibre, 0 mg chol, 200 mg sodium

Red Grape, Arugula and Toasted Walnut Salad

Walnut oil may be more expensive than olive oil or canola oil, but it's well worth the extra cost thanks to its exceptional ALA content (an omega-3 fat) and rich nutty flavour. Walnut oil can vary widely in flavour; for the best-tasting oil, look for a product that's unrefined.

Serves 6

Salad

1/2 cup (125 mL) coarsely chopped walnut halves

4 cups (1 L) tightly packed arugula

2 cups (500 mL) red grapes, halved

Dressing

4 tbsp (50 mL) walnut oil

2 tbsp (25 mL) freshly squeezed lemon juice

2 tsp (10 mL) agave nectar (syrup)

1 tsp (5 mL) whole-grain mustard

Preheat oven to 350°F (180°C).

Arrange walnuts on a baking sheet and place in the oven for 5 to 7 minutes, or until fragrant; remove from heat and cool.

In a large mixing bowl, toss together arugula, grapes and toasted walnuts; set aside.

In a small mixing bowl, whisk together walnut oil, lemon juice, agave nectar and mustard.

Drizzle dressing over salad; serve immediately.

TIP: Walnut oil is susceptible to damage from heat and light and has a limited shelf life. Keep it in a cool, dark place or in the refrigerator for up to 6 months.

Per 1 cup (250 mL) salad and 1 tbsp (15 mL) dressing: 182 cal, 2 g pro, 15 g total fat (1 g saturated fat), 13 g carb, 1 g fibre, 0 mg chol, 15 mg sodium

Roasted Beet Salad

Beets are an excellent source of anthocyanins, antioxidants that can help keep your heart healthy. This colourful salad takes a little longer to prepare than most of the salad recipes in this book, but the end result is well worth the time and effort.

Serves 4

4 medium-sized beets

1/2 cup (125 mL) chopped red onion

2 tbsp (25 mL) seasoned rice vinegar

1/2 tbsp (7 mL) Dijon mustard

1 tsp (5 mL) extra virgin olive oil

2 green onions, finely sliced

1 tsp (5 mL) orange zest

Preheat oven to 375°F (190°C).

Trim beets and cut into quarters.

Place beets in a glass baking dish; cover with 1/2 cup (125 mL) water. Cover baking dish with foil; bake for 50 to 60 minutes or until beets are tender. (Keep an eye on the beets while they are baking; if the bottom of the dish dries out, add another 1/2 cup/125 mL of water.)

Remove from heat and cool.

When beets are cool enough to handle, peel and dice them.

In a large bowl, combine diced beets, red onion, rice vinegar, mustard, olive oil, green onion and orange zest. Toss to coat.

Per 3/4 cup (175 mL) serving: 60 cal, 2 g pro, 1 g total fat (0 g saturated fat), 11 g carb, 2 g fibre, 0 mg chol, 121 mg sodium

Sesame Coleslaw

The sesame oil and rice wine vinegar in this recipe turn regular coleslaw into a flavourful, Asian-inspired salad. I suggest making it a day in advance to allow the cabbage to marinate and soften in the dressing.

Serves 6

6 cups (1.5 L) shredded green or Savoy cabbage (about 1/2 medium head of cabbage)

1 1/2 cups (375 mL) shredded carrot

2 green onions, thinly sliced

1/4 cup (50 mL) seasoned rice wine vinegar

2 tbsp (25 mL) dark sesame oil

1 tsp (5 mL) granulated sugar

1 tsp (5 mL) mustard seeds

In a large bowl, combine cabbage, carrot and green onion.

In a small bowl, whisk together rice wine vinegar, sesame oil, sugar and mustard seeds. Drizzle over cabbage mixture. Toss to mix thoroughly.

Cover and refrigerate for at least 3 hours before serving.

TIP: This salad tastes better the longer it is allowed to sit, so make it a few hours or up to a day before you plan to serve it.

Per 1 1/4 cup (300 mL) serving: 89 cal, 2 g pro, 5 g total fat (1 g saturated fat), 11 g carb, 4 g fibre, 0 mg chol, 39 mg sodium

Spinach Salad with Strawberries, Pine Nuts and Champagne Vinaigrette

This is such an easy salad to prepare, and it is sure to impress your dinner guests. Other toasted nuts can be substituted for the pine nuts, including sliced almonds and shelled pistachios. You can also swap the spinach with another mild, leafy green, such as mesclun mix, or use half spinach and half arugula for a peppery version.

Serves 4

1/4 cup (50 mL) pine nuts

8 cups (2 L) baby spinach

2 cups (500 mL) sliced strawberries

1/4 cup (50 mL) thinly sliced red onion

2 tbsp (25 mL) extra virgin olive oil

2 tbsp (25 mL) champagne vinegar

4 tsp (20 mL) agave nectar (syrup)

1/2 tsp (2 mL) grainy Dijon mustard

Preheat oven to 350°F (180°C).

Arrange pine nuts on a baking sheet; bake for 5 to 7 minutes, or until pine nuts are light golden brown and fragrant. Remove from heat and set aside to cool.

In a large salad bowl, toss together spinach, strawberries and red onion.

In a small mixing bowl, whisk together olive oil, vinegar, agave nectar and mustard.

Sprinkle toasted pine nuts over salad and drizzle with vinaigrette. Serve immediately.

TIP: Champagne vinegar is a light and mild vinegar that works well when paired with fresh fruit, as is the case in this salad. If you don't have champagne vinegar, you can substitute an equal amount of white wine vinegar or apple cider vinegar.

Per 2 1/2 cups (625 mL) salad and 1 1/2 tbsp (22 mL) dressing: 184 cal, 4 g pro, 13 g total fat (1 g saturated fat), 17 g carb, 2 g fibre, 0 mg chol, 162 mg sodium

Mains

Chickpea Curry

Serve this rich, fragrant curry with steamed rice or a piece of naan bread. You can substitute just about any protein-rich food for the chickpeas, including lentils or tofu.

Serves 6

1 tbsp (15 mL) canola oil

6 black peppercorns

6 cloves

2 cups (500 mL) chopped onion

3 cloves garlic, crushed

1 tbsp (15 mL) grated ginger root

2 cans (19 oz/540 mL each) chickpeas, drained and rinsed well

1 cup (250 mL) crushed tomatoes

1 cup (250 mL) water

2 tsp (10 mL) coriander

2 tsp (10 mL) cumin

1/2 tsp (2 mL) turmeric

1/4 tsp (1 mL) salt

1/8 tsp (0.5 mL) cayenne pepper, or to taste

1/4 cup (50 mL) chopped cilantro

Heat canola oil in a medium saucepan over high heat. When pan is hot, add peppercorns and cloves and reduce heat to medium; sauté for 20 seconds, or until fragrant. Add onion; sauté for 8 to 10 minutes. Add garlic and ginger; sauté for another minute.

Add chickpeas, tomatoes, water, coriander, cumin, turmeric, salt and cayenne pepper. Stir to combine. Cover and simmer for 20 minutes.

Sprinkle with cilantro before serving.

Per 1 cup (250 mL) serving: 235 cal, 11 g pro, 6 g total fat (2 g saturated fat), 38 g carb, 7 g fibre, 7 mg chol, 163 mg sodium

Chipotle Chili

This recipe uses dried chipotle chili pepper powder, which gives it a rich, smoky flavour. You can find it in the spice section of your local grocery store or gourmet food shop. Be sure to save some of this chili for leftovers—it's even tastier after it's been sitting in the fridge for a day.

Serves 8

1 tbsp (15 mL) canola oil

1 cup (250 mL) chopped onion

3 cloves garlic, crushed

1 1/2 cups (375 mL) chopped green pepper (about 1 large)

1 can (28 oz/796 mL) diced tomatoes

1 can (19 oz/540 mL) kidney beans, drained and rinsed well

1 can (19 oz/540 mL) chickpeas, drained and rinsed well

1 can (14 oz/398 mL) baked beans in tomato sauce

1 1/2 cups (375 mL) fresh or frozen corn kernels

2 tbsp (25 mL) molasses

2 tbsp (25 mL) white vinegar

1 tbsp (15 mL) cocoa powder

1/2 tsp (2 mL) dried chipotle chili pepper powder

Heat oil in a large saucepan over medium heat. When pan is hot, add onion and sauté about 8 to 10 minutes. Add garlic and green pepper; sauté another minute.

Add tomatoes, kidney beans, chickpeas, baked beans, corn, molasses, vinegar, cocoa powder and chipotle chili pepper powder. Cover and bring to a gentle boil over high heat; reduce and simmer for 30 minutes.

Per 1 cup (250 mL) serving: 275 cal, 12 g pro, 4 g total fat (1 g saturated fat), 54 g carb, 10 g fibre, 0 mg chol, 434 mg sodium

Falafel Wrap with Lemon Tahini Sauce

Falafels are patties made of ground chickpeas and are a staple in Middle Eastern cuisine. While sometimes eaten on their own, they are often stuffed in a pita with pickled vegetables and a creamy sauce made from tahini (sesame seed paste). Usually falafels are deep-fried, which gives them a lovely crunchy texture but also a lot of calories. This version uses just a tablespoon of oil for pan-frying, which results in a crispy texture without the added fat.

Serves 6

1 can (19 oz/540 mL) chickpeas, drained and rinsed well

3/4 cup (175 mL) coarsely chopped parsley

1/2 cup (125 mL) coarsely chopped onion

1/2 cup (125 mL) coarsely chopped cilantro

1/4 cup (50 mL) whole wheat breadcrumbs

1 tbsp (15 mL) ground flaxseed + 3 tbsp (45 mL) water (egg replacer)

2 cloves garlic

1 tsp (5 mL) ground cumin

1/4 tsp (1 mL) coarse sea salt

Pinch red pepper flakes, or to taste

1 tbsp (15 mL) canola oil

1/4 cup (50 mL) tahini

2 tsp (10 mL) freshly squeezed lemon juice

2 tbsp (25 mL) water

3 whole wheat or multigrain pitas (6 inch/15 cm each), cut in half and opened to form a pocket

2 cups (500 mL) coarsely chopped spinach

1 large tomato, sliced

Whisk together the ground flaxseed with water to make the egg replacer.

In a food processor, combine chickpeas, parsley, onion, cilantro, breadcrumbs, egg replacer, garlic, cumin, salt and red pepper flakes; pulse until ingredients are well blended.

Using clean hands, form the falafel dough into 12 uniformly sized balls. Gently press on each falafel to flatten it until it's about 2 inches (5 cm) across. Place falafel balls on a plate and set aside.

Heat oil in a large skillet over medium heat. When pan is hot, add falafel balls and cook for 4 minutes per side, or until falafels are golden brown.

In a small bowl, whisk together tahini, lemon juice and water; mix until just combined and runny (add an extra tablespoon of water if tahini thickens too much).

Stuff each pita half with two falafel balls, spinach and tomato; drizzle with 1 tbsp (25 mL) lemon tahini sauce. Serve immediately.

Per serving: 312 cal, 12 g pro, 10 g total fat (1 g saturated fat), 44 g carb, 7 g fibre, 0 mg chol, 389 mg sodium

Moroccan Chickpea Stew

This tasty stew shows up regularly on my fall and winter menus. I love its blend of savoury and sweet ingredients. It reminds me of the wonderful meals I enjoyed in Morocco.

Serves 6

1 tbsp (15 mL) canola oil

1 cup (250 mL) chopped onion

2 cloves garlic, crushed

2 cups (500 mL) cubed sweet potatoes

1 cup (250 mL) sliced carrots

1/2 cup (125 mL) chopped celery

1 can (19 oz/540 mL) chickpeas, drained and rinsed well

1 can (28 oz/796 mL) diced tomatoes

1/4 cup (50 mL) dried apricots, coarsely chopped

1/4 cup (50 mL) raisins

1 tsp (5 mL) cinnamon

1/2 tsp (2 mL) each ground ginger, turmeric and nutmeg

1 bay leaf

In a large saucepan, heat oil over medium heat. When pan is hot, add onion and sauté for 8 to 10 minutes. Add garlic and sauté for another minute.

Add sweet potatoes, carrots, celery, chickpeas, tomatoes, apricots, raisins, cinnamon, ginger, turmeric, nutmeg and bay leaf. Cover and bring to a boil; reduce heat and simmer for 45 minutes.

Serve warm.

Per 1 1/3 cup (325 mL) serving: 236 cal, 8 g pro, 4 g total fat (0 g saturated fat), 46 g carb, 7 g fibre, 0 mg chol, 368 mg sodium

Mushroom Lentil Patties

These patties are tasty on their own or served on a whole-grain bun with horseradish, fresh spinach leaves, sliced avocado and tomato slices. Although I usually use white button mushrooms, cremini or shiitake mushrooms also work well in this recipe.

Serves 4

1 tbsp (15 mL) canola oil

1 cup (250 mL) chopped onion

4 cups (1 L) thinly sliced mushrooms

2 tbsp (25 mL) balsamic vinegar

2 cups (500 mL) shredded carrot

1 1/2 cups (375 mL) cooked or canned brown lentils, drained and rinsed well

1/2 cup (125 mL) whole wheat breadcrumbs

1/2 cup (125 mL) rolled oats

1/4 cup (50 mL) ground flaxseed

1/4 cup (50 mL) slivered almonds, coarsely chopped

2 eggs, beaten

1 tbsp (15 mL) Dijon mustard

1/2 tsp (2 mL) coarse sea salt, or to taste

1/8 tsp (0.5 mL) cayenne pepper, or to taste

Freshly ground black pepper, to taste

Heat oil in a skillet over medium heat. Add onion and sauté for 8 to 10 minutes. Add mushrooms and sauté for another 8 to 10 minutes, or until all moisture from the mushrooms has evaporated and the pan begins to dry out. Transfer mushrooms and onion to a large mixing bowl.

Deglaze the skillet by pouring in the balsamic vinegar and scraping the bottom to lift up any onion or mushroom bits. Pour the vinegar mixture over the mushrooms.

Preheat oven to 350°F (180°C).

Add the carrot, lentils, breadcrumbs, oats, flaxseed, almonds, eggs, mustard, sea salt and cayenne pepper to the bowl. Stir until well combined with the mushrooms and onion. Season with black pepper.

Spray a baking sheet with cooking spray. With your hands, form mushroom and lentil mixture into 8 patties. Place on the baking sheet and bake for 20 to 25 minutes, or until they are cooked through and begin to brown.

Per 2 patties: 206 cal, 10 g pro, 8 g total fat (1 g saturated fat), 27 g carb, 6 g fibre, 37 mg chol, 260 mg sodium

Three Bean Garden Chili

This hearty meal is packed with fibre-rich legumes, providing 16 grams of fibre per serving. Cocoa and cinnamon give the chili a unique, subtle flavour that will leave your guests guessing at the secret ingredient that makes it taste so good. This chili is a breeze to make and freezes well.

Serves 8

1 tbsp (15 mL) canola oil

2 cups (500 mL) chopped onion

3 cloves garlic, crushed

1 1/2 cups (375 mL) diced red bell pepper

1 1/2 cups (375 mL) diced green bell pepper

2 cans (28 oz/796 mL each) diced tomatoes

1 can (19 oz/540 mL) kidney beans, drained and rinsed well

1 can (19 oz/540 mL) black beans, drained and rinsed well

1 can (19 oz/540 mL) chickpeas, drained and rinsed well

1 cup (250 mL) chopped carrot

1/2 cup (125 mL) corn kernels, fresh or frozen

2–3 tbsp (25–45 mL) chili powder

2 tbsp (25 mL) unsweetened cocoa

1/2 tsp (2 mL) cinnamon

1/4 tsp (1 mL) cayenne pepper, or to taste

2 tbsp (25 mL) tomato paste

Freshly ground black pepper, to taste

Heat oil in a large saucepan over medium heat. When pan is hot, add onion and sauté for 8 to 10 minutes. Add garlic and bell peppers and sauté for 2 to 3 minutes.

Add tomatoes, kidney beans, black beans, chickpeas, carrot, corn, chili powder, cocoa, cinnamon, cayenne pepper and tomato paste. Stir to combine. Season with black pepper. Cover and bring to a boil; reduce heat and simmer for 35 minutes.

Per 1 1/2 cup (375 mL) serving: 280 cal, 14 g pro, 4 g total fat (1 g saturated fat), 51 g carb, 13 g fibre, 0 mg chol, 375 mg sodium

Whole-Grain Lentil Casserole

I've been making this casserole for years and still love it. It's also become a huge hit with my clients—even kids like it! Serve it with steamed broccoli for a satisfying plant-based meal. I usually double this recipe so I have extra for lunches during the week.

Serves 4

1 1/2 cups (375 mL) sodium-reduced vegetable stock

1/2 cup (125 mL) dried green lentils

1/2 cup (125 mL) uncooked brown rice

1 cup (250 mL) stewed tomatoes

1/2 cup (125 mL) dry white wine or freshly squeezed lemon juice

1 cup (250 mL) chopped onion

1 clove garlic, crushed

1/4 tsp (1 mL) dried thyme

1/4 tsp (1 mL) dried basil

1 bay leaf

Freshly ground black pepper, to taste

1/2 cup (125 mL) shredded soy cheese (optional)

Preheat oven to 350°F (180°C).

In a 6 cup (1.5 L) casserole dish, combine stock, lentils, rice, tomatoes, wine, onion, garlic, thyme, basil, bay leaf and pepper.

Cover with foil and bake for 90 minutes, stirring 2 or 3 times. Sprinkle soy cheese on top and bake for another 5 minutes.

Per 1 1/2 cup (375 mL) serving: 288 cal, 15 g pro, 4 g total fat (0 g saturated fat), 43 g carb, 5 g fibre, 0 mg chol, 491 mg sodium

Balsamic Glazed Mushroom and Soy Burgers

These meat-free burgers contain texturized vegetable protein, a dehydrated meat alternative made from soybeans. Bob's Red Mill carries it in their line of dried goods and it's also available in the bulk section of most health food stores. The combination of sweet balsamic glazed mushrooms and nutty ground flaxseed makes for a delicious and healthy alternative to beef burgers. Taste-testers, including meat-lovers, couldn't get enough of these!

Serves 10

2 cups (500 mL) dry texturized vegetable protein granules, such as Bob's Red Mill

2 cups (500 mL) sodium-reduced vegetable stock

2 tbsp (25 mL) canola oil

2 cups (500 mL) chopped onion

3 cups (750 mL) sliced brown mushrooms, such as portobello or cremini

4 cloves garlic, crushed

2 tbsp (25 mL) balsamic vinegar

1 tbsp (15 mL) ground flaxseed + 3 tbsp (45 mL) water (egg replacer)

1/2 cup (125 mL) ground flaxseed

1/4 cup (50 mL) quick-cooking oats

1/4 cup (50 mL) whole wheat breadcrumbs

1/2 tsp (2 mL) red pepper flakes, or to taste

1/2 tsp (2 mL) coarse sea salt, or to taste

Freshly ground black pepper, to taste

1 tsp (5 mL) canola oil

Place texturized vegetable protein in a large mixing bowl.

In a saucepan, bring stock to a boil. Remove from heat and pour over texturized vegetable protein. Stir together until all of the liquid is absorbed. Set aside.

Heat 2 tbsp (25 mL) oil in a skillet over medium heat; add onion and mushrooms and sauté for 15 to 18 minutes, or until pan begins to dry out. Add garlic and sauté for another minute. Remove skillet from heat and drizzle with balsamic vinegar.

Add warm mushroom balsamic mixture to texturized vegetable protein and set aside to cool.

Meanwhile, make egg replacer by whisking together 1 tbsp of ground flaxseed with 3 tbsp water.

When texturized vegetable protein and mushroom mixture is cool, add egg replacer, ground flaxseed, oats, breadcrumbs, red pepper flakes, salt and pepper. Stir ingredients together until mixed well and mixture begins to hold its shape.

Use a 1/3-cup measure to scoop out mixture to form each burger. Firmly press ingredients together using your hands. Set formed burgers aside.

Heat 1 tsp (5 mL) oil in a skillet over medium heat. Add burgers and cook until brown and slightly crispy on the outside, about 5 to 6 minutes per side.

TIP: Serve these burgers in small whole-grain dinner rolls—or eat as open-faced sandwiches—topped with spinach, tomato, red onion slices and mashed avocado. To bake burgers instead, preheat oven to 375°F (190°C). Place burgers on a lightly oiled baking sheet and bake for 40 to 45 minutes, turning once, until they are cooked through.

Per burger: 174 cal, 14 g pro, 6 g total fat (1 g saturated fat), 16 g carb, 6 g fibre, 0 mg chol, 163 mg sodium

Grilled Tofu with Sautéed Greens

I often make this for vegetarian guests when hosting a barbecue, or when I feel like eating something lighter than a veggie burger. You can use other greens in place of the spinach, including bok choy or Swiss chard. If you don't have black sesame seeds, regular white sesame seeds work just as well.

Serves 2

Grilled Tofu

1 pkg (12 oz/350 g) extra-firm tofu

2 tsp (10 mL) sesame oil

2 tbsp (25 mL) unseasoned rice vinegar

1 tbsp (15 mL) brown sugar

1 clove garlic, crushed

Sautéed Greens

1 tsp (5 mL) canola oil

1 clove garlic, crushed

8 cups (2 L) baby spinach leaves

Pinch red pepper flakes, or to taste

Freshly ground black pepper, to taste

Pinch coarse sea salt, or to taste

1/4 tsp (1 mL) black sesame seeds

Slice tofu widthwise into 6 pieces (each slice about 3/4-inch thick).

Place a layer of paper towel, or a clean tea towel, on a cutting board. Arrange tofu in a single layer; cover with another layer of paper towel (or tea towel) and firmly press on tofu to remove excess moisture. Repeat two more times with dry paper towels or tea towels.

In a shallow dish, whisk together sesame oil, rice vinegar, brown sugar and garlic. Add tofu; marinate for at least 30 minutes, turning once.

Preheat grill over medium heat.

Meanwhile, heat canola oil in a skillet over medium heat. When pan is hot, add garlic and sauté for 30 seconds. Add spinach and sauté for 2 minutes, or until most of the spinach is wilted but some leaves still retain their shape. Season with red pepper flakes and pepper; remove from heat and cover to keep warm.

Place tofu on preheated grill and reduce heat to medium-low. Grill for 4 to 5 minutes per side, turning once or twice, or until tofu turns golden brown and has visible grill marks.

Divide sautéed greens between two plates; sprinkle with sea salt and black sesame seeds. Gently place three pieces of tofu over sautéed greens.

Serve immediately.

Per serving: 345 cal, 28 g pro, 20 g total fat (2 g saturated fat), 17 g carb, 0 g fibre, 0 mg chol, 442 mg sodium

Sesame Crusted Tofu

Although the tofu in this recipe needs marinating for only 1 hour, it's even more flavourful when marinated overnight. Enjoy these tofu cutlets on their own, in a burrito, or as a sandwich filling. I like to eat them in a sandwich made with whole-grain toast, avocado slices, Lemon Hummus (page 207), fresh basil, coarse sea salt and freshly ground black pepper.

Serves 2

2 tbsp (25 mL) sodium-reduced soy sauce

2 tbsp (25 mL) freshly squeezed lime juice

1 tsp (5 mL) sesame oil

2 cloves garlic, crushed

1 pkg (12 oz/350 g) extra-firm tofu, cut into 8 slices

1/4 cup (50 mL) sesame seeds

1 tbsp (15 mL) canola oil

In a small bowl, whisk together soy sauce, lime juice, sesame oil and garlic.

Lay tofu in a single layer in a glass baking dish. Pour soy sauce mixture over tofu and refrigerate for at least 1 hour.

Spread sesame seeds on a plate. Remove tofu from marinade 1 piece at a time and dredge in sesame seeds.

Heat oil in a skillet over high heat. Add tofu and reduce heat to medium-high; fry for 6 to 8 minutes per side, or until tofu begins to brown and gets crispy.

Per 4 slices of tofu: 421 cal, 29 g pro, 31 g total fat (4 g saturated fat), 12 g carb, 2 g fibre, 0 mg chol, 564 mg sodium

Spicy Baked Tofu

These spicy tofu bites are delicious served with a vegetable side, but they also make a great high-protein snack that even kids will enjoy!

Serves 2

3 tbsp (45 mL) sodium-reduced soy sauce

3 tbsp (45 mL) unseasoned rice vinegar

1 tbsp (15 mL) honey

2 cloves garlic, crushed

1 tsp (5 mL) sesame oil

1/4 tsp (1 mL) red pepper flakes

1 pkg (12 oz/350 g) extra-firm tofu, cut into 1-inch/2.5 cm cubes

In a shallow dish, combine soy sauce, vinegar, honey, garlic, sesame oil and red pepper flakes. Add tofu; cover and marinate in the fridge for a couple of hours or overnight.

Preheat oven to 350°F (180°C).

Remove tofu from marinade and place on a baking sheet.

Bake for 15 to 20 minutes or until tofu begins to brown.

Serve warm.

Per serving: 257 cal, 26 g pro, 14 g total fat (2 g saturated fat), 10 g carb, 0 g fibre, 0 mg chol, 429 mg sodium

Tempeh Vegetable Summer Rolls

Like tofu, tempeh is extremely versatile, taking on the flavour of
whatever it is cooked with. There are different types of tempeh,
including those made from quinoa and kasha. Any type can be
used in this recipe. These summer rolls taste great with other fresh
ingredients, such as sliced mango and basil leaves, so be creative.

Serves 6

Summer Rolls

1 block (8 1/2 oz/240 g) tempeh

1/2 pkg (8 oz/250 g) vermicelli noodles

1 tsp (5 mL) canola oil

2 cloves garlic, crushed

1 tbsp (15 mL) minced ginger root

1 tbsp (15 mL) sodium-reduced soy sauce

12 pieces (9 inch/23 cm each) rice paper

2 cups (500 mL) baby spinach leaves

1 cup (250 mL) shredded carrot

1 cup (250 mL) chopped cilantro

1 1/2 cups (375 mL) thinly sliced red pepper strips

1/2 cup (125 mL) coarsely chopped mint leaves

Hoisin Dipping Sauce

1/2 cup (125 mL) hoisin sauce

2 tbsp (25 mL) sweet chili sauce

Cut tempeh into 1/4-inch (5 mm) thick strips; set aside.

Fill a large saucepan with water and bring to a boil. When water begins to boil, remove from heat. Soak noodles in the water for 2 to 3 minutes, until they become soft; drain immediately and run under cold water.

Meanwhile, heat oil in a skillet over medium heat. Add garlic and ginger; sauté for 1 minute. Add tempeh and soy sauce; cook until tempeh is slightly crispy. Remove from heat and set aside.

Fill a large mixing bowl with lukewarm water. Add 1 piece of rice paper and gently move it around with your fingers until the paper is soft and flexible (about 30 seconds); immediately remove from water, gently shaking off any excess moisture. Lay the rice paper on a plate.

In the middle of the rice paper, arrange a small handful (about 1/4 cup/50 mL) of noodles and a sixth of the remaining ingredients, including tempeh, spinach, carrot, cilantro, red pepper and mint leaves. Gently fold the bottom of the rice paper over the filling. Holding it firmly in place, fold both sides of the wrapper toward the middle. Then, pressing firmly down to hold the folds in place, roll the entire pile upward to close the top. Seal any loose seams with a dab of water.

Place finished rolls on a clean plate; cover with a damp, clean tea towel or damp paper towels. Repeat the process with the remaining ingredients.

In a small bowl, combine hoisin sauce and sweet chili sauce.

Serve immediately.

Per 2 rolls: 275 cal, 10 g pro, 5 g total fat (1 g saturated fat), 48 g carb, 5 g fibre, 1 mg chol, 393 mg sodium

Per 2 rolls with 1 1/2 tbsp (22 mL) hoisin dipping sauce: 325 cal, 11 g pro, 6 g fat (1 g saturated fat), 58 g carb, 6 g fibre, 2 mg chol, 757 mg sodium

Quinoa Stuffed Red Bell Peppers

Pale yellow quinoa is the most widely available variety of this high-protein whole grain, though some natural food stores carry a dark reddish-brown variety. Both are prepared the same way. If you want a more colourful dish, use equal parts yellow and red quinoa.

Serves 6

6 small red bell peppers

1 tbsp (15 mL) canola oil

1/2 cup (125 mL) chopped onion

1 cup (250 mL) shredded carrot

3 cloves garlic, crushed

2 cups (500 mL) cooked quinoa

2 tbsp (25 mL) chopped chives

1 tbsp (15 mL) chopped fresh basil

2 tbsp (25 mL) freshly squeezed lemon juice or vegetable broth

Preheat oven to 375°F (190°C).

Cut off and reserve the tops of the bell peppers. Scoop out and discard the ribs and seeds.

Heat canola oil in a skillet over medium heat. Add onion and carrot and sauté until onion is translucent, about 5 minutes. Add garlic; sauté for another minute. Remove from heat.

In a large bowl, combine quinoa, onion mixture, chives, basil and lemon juice. Stuff each pepper with the quinoa mixture, evenly distributing the mixture among the peppers. Place a reserved top on each of the peppers.

Gently place the peppers in a glass baking dish. Bake for 30 minutes. If the peppers begin to burn on the bottom, add about 1/2 cup (125 mL) water to the baking dish.

Per stuffed pepper: 296 cal, 10 g pro, 6 g total fat (0 g saturated fat), 54 g carb, 7 g fibre, 0 mg chol, 21 mg sodium

Vegetable Sides

Balsamic Swiss Chard

Swiss chard is one of my favourite leafy green vegetables—it's a side I serve often. Swiss chard with pale green stems is the most common type you'll find in grocery stores. But you can also find ruby chard, with brightly coloured red stems. At farmers' markets during the summer you may also see rainbow chard, a mix of Swiss chard, ruby chard and golden chard. If you grow Swiss chard in your garden, double or triple this recipe and freeze the leftovers so you can enjoy it throughout the winter months.

Serves 4

1 tsp (5 mL) canola oil

2 cloves garlic, crushed

6 cups (1.5 L) chard (Swiss, rainbow or ruby), washed and trimmed

1 tbsp (15 mL) balsamic vinegar

1/4 tsp (1 mL) coarse sea salt

Freshly ground black pepper, to taste

Heat oil in a skillet over medium heat. Add garlic and sauté for 1 minute. Add Swiss chard; cover and steam for 4 to 5 minutes, until chard begins to wilt.

Remove from heat and sprinkle with vinegar. Season with salt and pepper.

Per serving: 23 cal, 1 g pro, 1 g total fat (0 g saturated fat), 3 g carb, 1 g fibre, 0 mg chol, 266 mg sodium

Broccoli with Sesame Dressing

The combination of rice vinegar, sesame oil, ginger root and sesame seeds is a perfect match for broccoli. When sautéing the broccoli, be careful not to overcook it—it should be slightly crunchy.

Serves 6

1 tsp (5 mL) canola oil

3 cloves garlic, crushed

3 cups (750 mL) broccoli, cut into bite-sized pieces

1 tbsp (15 mL) rice vinegar

1 tbsp (15 mL) dark sesame oil

1 tsp (5 mL) chopped ginger root

1 tbsp (15 mL) sesame seeds

Heat oil in a skillet over medium heat. Add garlic and broccoli; sauté until garlic is fragrant and broccoli is tender, about 4 to 5 minutes.

Transfer broccoli to a large bowl; set aside to cool.

Meanwhile, in a small bowl, whisk together rice vinegar, sesame oil and ginger. Drizzle over broccoli. Sprinkle sesame seeds on top. Serve warm or cold.

TIP: Look for a brand of rice vinegar with less than 60 mg of sodium per tablespoon (15 mL) to keep the sodium down.

Per serving: 127 cal, 10 g pro, 5 g total fat (1 g saturated fat), 18 g carb, 8 g fibre, 0 mg chol, 86 mg sodium

Garlic Roasted Cauliflower

If you're looking for a new way to cook cauliflower, look no farther. Roasting the cauliflower gives it a delicious nutty flavour and crispy texture. I like to use plenty of freshly ground black pepper to give the cauliflower extra spice.

Serves 4

1 medium cauliflower, cut into bite-sized pieces (about 4 cups/1 L)

1 tbsp (15 mL) canola oil

1 clove garlic, crushed

1/4 tsp (1 mL) coarse sea salt

Freshly ground black pepper, to taste

Preheat oven to 375°F (190°C).

In a large bowl, toss together cauliflower, oil, garlic, salt and pepper.

Spread cauliflower mixture on a baking sheet. Bake for 22 to 25 minutes, or until edges begin to brown and the cauliflower is tender-crisp when pierced with a fork.

Per serving: 68 cal, 3 g pro, 4 g total fat (1 g saturated fat), 8 g carb, 3 g fibre, 0 mg chol, 190 mg sodium

Grilled Balsamic Portobello Mushrooms

Portobello mushrooms have a meaty texture and rich flavour, making them a delicious vegetarian alternative to a steak or beef burger. I also like to add these mushrooms to a platter of mixed grilled vegetables—they're delicious. In fact, you may want to grill extra for lunch the next day.

Serves 4

4 portobello mushrooms, washed and trimmed

1 tbsp (15 mL) olive oil

1 tbsp (15 mL) balsamic vinegar

1/4 tsp (1 mL) coarse sea salt

Freshly cracked pepper, to taste

Preheat grill over medium heat.

In a bowl, toss mushrooms with olive oil, vinegar, salt and pepper.

Place mushrooms on grill; cook for 4 to 5 minutes, turning once or twice, or until mushrooms begin to brown.

Per grilled mushroom: 55 cal, 2 g pro, 4 g total fat (1 g saturated fat), 5 g carb, 1 g fibre, 0 mg chol, 152 mg sodium

Maple Dijon Carrots

This quick side dish rich in beta-carotene feeds a crowd. If you're a mustard fan, try making this recipe with different variations of mustard, such as whole grain or honey Dijon.

Serves 8

4 cups (1 L) sliced carrots, medallions

1 tbsp (15 mL) maple syrup

1 tsp (5 mL) Dijon mustard

Freshly ground black pepper, to taste

Fill a medium saucepan with water. Add carrots and bring to a boil. Reduce heat and simmer until carrots are tender, about 8 to 10 minutes.

Drain carrots. Stir in maple syrup and mustard until well combined. Season with black pepper.

Per 1/2 cup (125 mL) serving: 55 cal, 1 g pro, 0 g total fat (0 g saturated fat), 13 g carb, 3 g fibre, 0 mg chol, 44 mg sodium

Lemon Swiss Chard

I love to serve Swiss chard with a little lemon juice—it really brings
out the flavour of the chard. To amp up the flavour, I sometimes like to
add a little grated lemon zest before serving.

Serves 4

1 tsp (5 mL) canola oil

1 clove garlic, crushed

6 cups (1.5 L) Swiss chard, washed and trimmed

1 tbsp (15 mL) lemon juice

1/4 tsp (1 mL) coarse sea salt, or to taste

Freshly ground black pepper, to taste

In a large skillet, heat oil over medium heat. Add garlic and sauté for
1 minute.

Add Swiss chard; cover and steam for several minutes, until the chard
is wilted.

Remove from heat and sprinkle with lemon juice, salt and pepper.
Serve warm.

Per serving: 22 cal, 1 g pro, 1 g total fat (0 g saturated fat), 2 g carb,
1 g fibre, 0 mg chol, 266 mg sodium

Oven Roasted Brussels Sprouts

If your family members turn up their noses at Brussels sprouts, I think this recipe will change their opinion. It's the way I serve them most often because they taste so great. Roasting Brussels sprouts mellows their earthy flavour—they taste almost like an entirely different vegetable.

Serves 4

4 cups (1 L) Brussels sprouts, halved, ends trimmed

1 1/2 tbsp (22 mL) olive oil

1/2 tsp (2 mL) coarse sea salt

Freshly ground black pepper, to taste

Preheat oven to 400°F (200°C).

In a bowl, toss Brussels sprouts with oil, salt and pepper.

Transfer to a baking sheet lined with parchment paper. Bake for 20 to 25 minutes, or until Brussels sprouts are golden brown and tender when pierced with a fork.

TIP: Cooking time depends largely on the size of the sprouts, so keep an eye on them. They're done when they can be pierced easily with a fork and start to get brown and crispy around the edges.

Per serving: 83 cal, 3 g pro, 5 g total fat (1 g saturated fat), 8 g carb, 4 g fibre, 0 mg chol, 168 mg sodium

Roasted Gingered Squash

Roasting the squash with ginger root and orange zest adds plenty of flavour. It's a delicious way to get your beta-carotene.

Serves 4

2 cups (500 mL) butternut squash (about 1 medium squash)

2 tbsp (25 mL) grated ginger root

2 tbsp (25 mL) agave nectar (syrup)

1 tbsp (15 mL) orange zest

1 tbsp (15 mL) olive oil

1/4 tsp (1 mL) coarse sea salt

Preheat oven to 375°F (190°C).

Cut squash into 1-inch (2.5 cm) cubes. In a large bowl, toss squash with ginger, agave nectar, orange zest, oil and salt.

Spread squash on a baking sheet and bake for 30 to 40 minutes, or until tender.

Per serving: 96 cal, 1 g pro, 4 g total fat (1 g saturated fat), 17 g carb, 1 g fibre, 0 mg chol, 150 mg sodium

Simple Sautéed Spinach with Lemon

Spinach gets two thumbs up when it comes to nutrition. It's high in vitamin C, vitamin K, folate, iron, magnesium and potassium and low in calories. And it's loaded with lutein, an antioxidant that helps keep your eyes healthy as you age.

Serves 4

1 tbsp (15 mL) olive oil

2 cloves garlic, crushed

8 cups (2 L) spinach

2 tbsp (25 mL) freshly squeezed lemon juice

1/4 tsp (1 mL) coarse sea salt, or to taste

Freshly ground black pepper, to taste

Pinch red pepper flakes, or to taste

Heat oil in a large skillet over medium heat. Add garlic and sauté for 1 minute.

Add spinach, lemon juice, salt, pepper and red pepper flakes to skillet; cover and steam for 3 to 4 minutes, or until spinach is wilted. Remove from heat and serve immediately.

Per serving: 60 cal, 3 g pro, 4 g total fat (1 g saturated fat), 5 g carb, 3 g fibre, 0 mg chol, 236 mg sodium

Spicy Sautéed Kale

With its unmistakable dark green curly leaves, kale is as attractive as it is nutritious. Gram for gram, kale outshines most other leafy green vegetables when it comes to vitamins A, C, E and K. This recipe is a great way to introduce the leafy green vegetable into your diet if you're not familiar with it.

Serves 4

1 tbsp (15 mL) olive oil

2 cloves garlic, crushed

8 cups (2 L) kale, stems removed, washed, trimmed and torn into bite-sized pieces

1/3 cup (75 mL) water

1 tbsp (15 mL) red wine vinegar

1/4 tsp (1 mL) red pepper flakes, or to taste

1/4 tsp (1 mL) coarse sea salt, or to taste

Freshly ground black pepper, to taste

Heat oil in a large skillet over medium heat. Add garlic and sauté for 1 minute.

Add kale, water, red wine vinegar, red pepper flakes, salt and pepper to skillet.

Cover and steam for 10 to 12 minutes, or until kale is wilted and tender.

Remove from heat and serve immediately.

Per serving: 100 cal, 5 g pro, 4 g total fat (1 g saturated fat), 14 g carb, 3 g fibre, 0 mg chol, 205 mg sodium

Spinach with Spicy Peanut Sauce

The peanut sauce in this recipe tastes wonderful on spinach, but it can also be used on grilled vegetables. Or try it as a dipping sauce for Tempeh Vegetable Summer Rolls (page 191).

Serves 4

1 tsp (5 mL) canola oil

2 cloves garlic, crushed

1 tbsp (15 mL) grated ginger root

8 cups (2 L) spinach

2 tbsp (25 mL) peanut butter

2 tsp (10 mL) freshly squeezed lime juice

1 tsp (5 mL) sodium-reduced soy sauce

Pinch cayenne pepper, or to taste

Heat oil in a large skillet over medium heat. When skillet is hot, add garlic and ginger and sauté for 1 minute. Add spinach, cover pan and let steam for 2 to 3 minutes until wilted.

Meanwhile, in a small bowl, whisk together peanut butter, lime juice, soy sauce and cayenne pepper.

When spinach is just wilted, remove from heat and drizzle with peanut sauce. Serve immediately.

Per serving: 88 cal, 5 g pro, 6 g total fat (1 g saturated fat), 7 g carb, 4 g fibre, 0 mg chol, 168 mg sodium

Snacks

Black Bean Hummus

Hummus has a long history in the Middle East, where it is traditionally made with chickpeas. This version uses black beans instead. Gram for gram, black beans have 15 percent more fibre and 25 percent fewer calories than chickpeas. And they beat out other beans when it comes to antioxidants. This hummus is a delicious dip for vegetables and also makes a tasty spread on whole-grain crackers.

Serves 8

1 can (19 oz/540 mL) black beans, drained and rinsed well

1/4 cup (50 mL) tahini

3 tbsp (45 mL) freshly squeezed lemon juice

2 tbsp (25 mL) olive oil

1 clove garlic, crushed

1/8 tsp (0.5 mL) red pepper flakes, or to taste

1 tbsp (15 mL) finely chopped parsley (optional)

In a food processor, combine black beans, tahini, lemon juice, olive oil, garlic and red pepper flakes; pulse until smooth, or desired consistency. Alternatively, use the back of a fork to mash ingredients until smooth, or desired consistency.

Place in a serving bowl and garnish with fresh parsley. Serve cold or at room temperature.

Per 1/4 cup (50 mL) serving: 130 cal, 5 g pro, 8 g total fat (1 g saturated fat), 12 g carb, 3 g fibre, 0 mg chol, 3 mg sodium

Kale Chips with Sea Salt

These yummy "chips" are a far healthier alternative to potato chips and provide an easy way to boost your intake of leafy green vegetables. Kale is an excellent source of beta-carotene and one serving of these chips provides more than a day's worth of vitamins C and K. Kale's sturdy leaves are ideally suited to making these crispy chips. I suggest making extra—they won't last long!

Serves 4

4 cups (1 L) kale, washed, trimmed and torn into bite-sized pieces

1 tbsp (15 mL) olive oil

1/2 tsp (2 mL) sea salt

Freshly ground black pepper, to taste

Preheat oven to 350°F (180°C).

In a large mixing bowl, toss together kale, olive oil, salt and pepper. Use clean hands to gently rub the oil into the kale.

Spread kale on a large baking sheet. Bake for 15 minutes, or until kale is crispy.

Cool and serve.

Per 1 cup (250 mL) serving: 63 cal, 2 g pro, 4 g total fat (1 g saturated fat), 7 g carb, 2 g fibre, 0 mg chol, 321 mg sodium

Lemon Hummus

This creamy hummus is a crowd-pleaser—serve it with carrot sticks or whole-grain crackers at parties and get-togethers. It also makes for a tasty spread on soy burgers and sandwiches, especially when paired with sliced tomatoes and baby spinach leaves.

Serves 6

1 can (19 oz/540 mL) chickpeas, drained and rinsed well

1/3 cup (75 mL) tahini

1/4 cup (50 mL) freshly squeezed lemon juice

2 tbsp (25 mL) extra virgin olive oil

1 tbsp (15 mL) water

1/4 tsp (1 mL) coarse sea salt

In a food processor or blender, combine chickpeas, tahini, lemon juice, olive oil, water and salt; pulse to a smooth consistency.

Makes 1 1/2 cups (375 mL).

Per 1/4 cup (50 mL) serving: 205 cal, 7 g pro, 13 g total fat (2 g saturated fat), 18 g carb, 4 g fibre, 0 mg chol, 117 mg sodium

Sesame Ginger Edamame

While often served at Japanese restaurants as an appetizer, edamame is a quick and easy dish to make at home. I like to keep a few bags of edamame in the freezer for a satisfying snack—they are a great alternative to potato chips and popcorn.

Serves 4

1 1/2 tbsp (22 mL) sesame seeds

1 bag (1.1 lb/500 g) frozen edamame

1 tbsp (15 mL) grated ginger root

2 tsp (10 mL) sesame oil

1/2 tsp (2 mL) coarse sea salt, or to taste

Preheat oven to 350°F (180°C).

Place sesame seeds on a baking sheet. Bake for 5 to 7 minutes, or until seeds begin to brown and become fragrant; remove from heat and set aside.

Meanwhile, bring a saucepan full of water to a boil. Add edamame and cook for 4 to 5 minutes. Remove from heat and drain water.

In a mixing bowl, toss edamame with ginger, sesame oil, salt and toasted sesame seeds.

Serve warm.

TIP: Swap regular sesame seeds for black sesame seeds, available at major grocery and specialty food stores, for an attractive variation.

Per 1 cup (250 mL) serving: 178 cal, 13 g pro, 10 g total fat (1 g saturated fat), 12 g carb, 6 g fibre, 0 mg chol, 300 mg sodium

Spicy Candied Walnuts

Sweet, salty and spicy—these walnuts have it all! Although this recipe makes an addictive cocktail snack year-round, it's also a special treat for holiday parties.

Serves 6

1 1/2 cups (375 mL) walnut halves

1/4 cup (50 mL) shredded unsweetened coconut

2 tbsp (25 mL) agave nectar (syrup)

1/8 tsp (0.5 mL) cayenne pepper, or to taste

Pinch salt, or to taste

1/3 cup (75 mL) dried cranberries

Preheat oven to 350°F (180°C).

In a medium bowl, combine walnuts, coconut, agave nectar, cayenne pepper and salt.

Spread walnut mixture onto a baking sheet and bake, turning once, for 8 to 10 minutes, or until brown and slightly crispy.

Transfer walnut mixture to a bowl to cool. Toss with cranberries. Store in an airtight container.

Per 1/4 cup (50 mL) serving: 251 cal, 8 g pro, 19 g total fat (2 g saturated fat), 18 g carb, 2 g fibre, 0 mg chol, 59 mg sodium

Tamari Roasted Almonds

These almonds take only minutes to prepare and are a tasty variation on regular toasted almonds. Add lemon zest for extra flavour.

Serves 6

1 1/2 cups (375 mL) raw unsalted almonds

2 tbsp (25 mL) tamari or sodium-reduced soy sauce

2 tbsp (25 mL) freshly squeezed lemon juice

Heat a skillet over medium heat. Add almonds and cook for 3 to 5 minutes, shaking skillet frequently, until nuts become fragrant.

Drizzle tamari and lemon juice over almonds and remove from heat as soon as pan begins to dry out.

Serve warm, or transfer almonds to a bowl to cool and then store in an airtight container.

Per 1/4 cup (50 mL) serving: 214 cal, 8 g pro, 18 g total fat (1 g saturated fat), 8 g carb, 4 g fibre, 0 mg chol, 171 mg sodium

Zesty Edamame

You'll find bags of edamame—frozen soybeans in pods—in the freezer section of most grocery stores and health food stores. They're nutritious and a quick snack to prepare; they need only be boiled for a few minutes and they're ready to enjoy. Best of all, kids love them, too!

Serves 4

1 bag (1.1 lb/500 g) frozen edamame

Zest of 1 lemon

1/2 tsp (2 mL) coarse sea salt, or to taste

1/8 tsp (0.5 mL) red pepper flakes

Fill a saucepan with water and bring to a boil. Add edamame and return water to a boil. Continue to boil for 3 to 4 minutes, then remove from heat and drain.

Place edamame in a serving bowl and toss with lemon zest, salt and red pepper flakes. Serve warm.

Per 1 cup (250 mL) serving: 138 cal, 13 g pro, 6 g total fat (0 g saturated fat), 11 g carb, 6 g fibre, 0 mg chol, 300 mg sodium

Desserts

Apple Raspberry Crisp with Maple Oat Topping

This recipe is delicious made with a variety of seasonal fruit. Try locally grown peaches or pears in place of apples, and blueberries or strawberries in place of raspberries.

Serves 6

1/2 cup (125 mL) whole wheat flour

3/4 cup (175 mL) rolled oats

1/2 cup (125 mL) oat bran

1 tsp (5 mL) cinnamon

1 tsp (5 mL) ground cloves

1 tsp (5 mL) vanilla extract

3 tbsp (45 mL) maple syrup

2 tbsp (25 mL) canola oil

8 cups (2 L) peeled and sliced apples

1 cup (250 mL) raspberries

Preheat oven to 375°F (190°C).

In a large bowl, combine flour, oats, oat bran, cinnamon, cloves, vanilla, maple syrup and oil. Mix until crumbly.

In an 8 × 8 inch (2 L) glass baking dish, combine apples and raspberries. Sprinkle crumble mixture over fruit.

Bake for 40 to 50 minutes or until fruit is soft and the top begins to brown.

TIP: Double the recipe for the crumble topping and freeze half in a resealable freezer bag. When you want to make this recipe, all you have to do is slice the fruit and add the topping directly from the freezer.

Per serving: 235 cal, 5 g pro, 7 g total fat (1 g saturated fat), 45 g carb, 7 g fibre, 0 mg chol, 3 mg sodium

Chocolate Fruit Fondue

Chocolate fondue recipes usually call for heavy cream, a source of cholesterol-raising saturated fat. This version skips the cream, making it slightly thicker but considerably lower in saturated fat. While the recipe calls for plain dark chocolate, you can also use specialty dark chocolate bars such as orange, mint, espresso or green tea. Buy dark chocolate with at least 70 percent cocoa solids: The higher the cocoa solids, the greater the concentration of antioxidants that may help keep blood pressure in check.

Serves 4

1 cup (250 mL) finely chopped dark chocolate (about 5 oz/140 g)

4 cups (1 L) mixed fresh fruit (such as strawberries, mango, apples, banana, kiwi or pineapple), cut into 1-inch/2.5-cm chunks

Using a double boiler (see Tip) and stirring constantly, melt chocolate until warm and smooth.

Remove from heat and pour into a heat-resistant bowl. Serve immediately with fresh fruit for dipping.

TIP: A double boiler is two saucepans that stack on top of each other. The bottom saucepan is filled with simmering water, while the top saucepan is filled with food that is cooked, or in this case melted, by the heat from below. If you don't have a double boiler, make your own: In a small saucepan, bring 1 to 2 inches (2.5 to 5 cm) of water to a boil, then place a stainless steel bowl over the mouth of the saucepan to hold the chocolate.

Per serving: 302 cal, 5 g pro, 18 g total fat (10 g saturated fat), 44 g carb, 4 g fibre, 0 mg chol, 4 mg sodium

Cinnamon Pecan Baked Apples

Baked apples conjure up thoughts of cool autumn days; however, these apples can be enjoyed year-round. It's important to use a firm variety of apple that will hold its shape after cooking, such as Spy or Idared.

Serves 4

4 apples

1/4 cup (50 mL) brown sugar

1 tbsp (15 mL) chopped pecans

1 tsp (5 mL) cinnamon

1 tbsp (15 mL) dried cranberries

1/2 tsp (1 mL) vanilla extract

Preheat oven to 375°F (190°C).

Using an apple corer, remove most of the apple core from each apple, leaving about 1/2 inch (1 cm) at the bottom.

In a small bowl, combine sugar, pecans, cinnamon, cranberries and vanilla.

Place the apples in a glass baking dish.

Place equal portions of sugar mixture in the hollow centre of each apple.

Cover the bottom of the dish with 1/4 inch (0.5 cm) of water.

Bake for 40 to 50 minutes, or until apples are soft but still hold their shape.

Per baked apple: 166 cal, 1 g pro, 3 g total fat (0 g saturated fat), 37 g carb, 3 g fibre, 0 mg chol, 6 mg sodium

Fresh Berries with Chocolate and Toasted Coconut

This easy-to-prepare dessert is the perfect way to showcase fresh, locally grown berries when they're in season during the summer. Toasted coconut, grated dark chocolate and a hint of lemon zest are the ultimate accompaniment to sweet, succulent berries. Feel free to swap other fresh berries for the strawberries, raspberries or blueberries, such as blackberries or Saskatoon berries—a dark purple berry native to western Canada.

Serves 4

1/3 cup (75 mL) unsweetened shredded coconut

2 cups (500 mL) quartered strawberries

1 cup (250 mL) fresh raspberries

1 cup (250 mL) fresh blueberries

1 tsp (5 mL) grated lemon zest

3–4 tbsp (45–50 g) dark chocolate, grated

Preheat oven to 350°F (180°C).

Place coconut on a baking sheet; bake for 5 to 7 minutes until light golden brown and fragrant. Remove from heat and cool.

Meanwhile, in a large bowl, toss together strawberries, raspberries, blueberries and lemon zest. Add coconut and combine until fruit is coated with coconut. Garnish with grated chocolate.

Serve immediately.

TIP: Use dark chocolate with at least 70% cocoa solids to get more antioxidants.

Per 1 cup (250 mL) serving: 160 cal, 2 g pro, 8 g total fat (7 g saturated fat), 23 g carb, 6 g fibre, 0 mg chol, 15 mg sodium

Tropical Fruit Salad with Lemon Maple Glaze

This recipe works well with just about any kind of fresh fruit, including fresh berries, grapes and orange segments. It's a simple and healthy way to end a meal and doesn't take much time to prepare. It also doubles as a delicious dish to serve at brunch. The fruit tastes even better after sitting in the marinade overnight, so make it in advance if you have time.

Serves 4

1/4 cup (50 mL) maple syrup

1/4 cup (50 mL) freshly squeezed lemon juice

2 cups (500 mL) diced mango

1 cup (250 mL) sliced kiwi

1 cup (250 mL) diced pineapple

4 mint leaves

Combine maple syrup and lemon juice in saucepan; bring to a boil over high heat. Boil for 3 minutes. Remove from heat and cool.

In a large bowl, toss together mango, kiwi and pineapple. Drizzle with cooled lemon maple glaze and garnish with mint leaves. Serve immediately.

Per 1 cup (250 mL) fruit with 1 tbsp (15 mL) glaze: 156 cal, 1 g pro, 1 g total fat (0 g saturated fat), 40 g carb, 3 g fibre, 0 mg chol, 5 mg sodium

References

Step 1

1. Heart and Stroke Foundation. Statistics. 2012. Available at www.heartandstroke.com/site/c.ikIQLcMWJtE/b.3483991/k.34A8/Statistics.htm
2. Canadian Diabetes Association. *Diabetes: Canada at the Tipping Point: Charting a New Path*. 2010. Available at www.diabetes.ca/documents/get-involved/WEB_Eng.CDA_Report_.pdf
3. Public Health Agency of Canada. *Obesity in Canada*. Available at www.phac-aspc.gc.ca/hp-ps/hl-mvs/oic-oac/index-eng.php
4. Canadian Cancer Society. *Canadian Cancer Statistics 2012*. Available at www.cancer.ca/Canada-wide/About%20cancer/Cancer%20statistics.aspx?sc_lang=en
5. Osteoporosis Canada. Facts and statistics. 2011. Available at www.osteoporosis.ca/index.php/ci_id/8867/la_id/1.htm=
6. Alzheimer Society of Canada. Fact sheets. 2012. Available at www.alzheimer.ca/en/%7E/~/media/Files/national/Core-lit-brochures/asc_factsheets_2012_e.ashx

Step 2

1. Fraser GE. Vegetarian diets: what do we know of their effects on common chronic diseases? *American Journal of Clinical Nutrition* 89(5):1607S–1612S, 2009.
2. Pettersen BJ, Anousheh R, Fan J et al. Vegetarian diets and blood pressure among white subjects: results from the Adventist Health Study–2 (AHS–2). *Public Health Nutrition* 10:1–8, 2012.
3. Rizzo NS, Sabate J, Jaceldo-Siegl K and Fraser GE. Vegetarian dietary patterns are associated with a lower risk of metabolic syndrome: the Adventist Health Study 2. *Diabetes Care* 34(5):1225–1227, 2011.
4. Esselstyn CB Jr, Ellis SG, Medendorp SV and Crowe TD. A strategy to arrest and reverse coronary artery disease: a 5-year longitudinal study of a single physician's practice. *Journal of Family Practice* 41(6):560–568, 1995.

5. Tonstad S, Stewart K, Oda K et al. Vegetarian diets and the incidence of diabetes in the Adventist Health Study–2. *Nutrition, Metabolism & Cardiovascular Diseases*, October 7, 2011 [epub ahead of print].

6. Tonstad S, Butler T, Yan R and Fraser GE. Type of vegetarian diet, body weight, and prevalence of type 2 diabetes. *Diabetes Care* 32(5):791–796, 2009.

7. Barnard ND, Cohen J, Jenkins DJ et al. A low-fat vegan diet and a conventional diabetes diet in the treatment of type 2 diabetes: a randomized, controlled, 74-wk clinical trial. *American Journal of Clinical Nutrition* 89(5):1588S–1596S, 2009.

8. Singh PN, Sebate J and Fraser GE. Does low meat consumption increase life expectancy in humans? *American Journal of Clinical Nutrition* 78(3 Suppl):526S–532S, 2003.

9. Key TJ, Appleby PN, Davey GK et al. Mortality in British vegetarians: review and preliminary results from EPIC-Oxford. *American Journal of Clinical Nutrition* 78(3 Suppl):533S–538S, 2003.

10. World Society for the Protection of Animals. *What's on your plate? The hidden costs of industrial animal agriculture in Canada.* Toronto, 2012.

11. Ibid.

12. Michael Pollan. Profiles in courage on animal welfare. *The New York Times*, May 29, 2006. Available at http://pollan.blogs.nytimes.com/2006/05/29/profiles-in-courage-on-animal-welfare/

Step 3

1. Vallejo F, Tomás-Barberán FA, and García-Viguera C. Phenolic compound contents in edible parts of broccoli inflorescences after domestic cooking. *Journal of the Science of Food and Agriculture* 83(14):1511–1516, 2003.

2. Halvorsen BL, Carlsen MH, Phillips KM et al. Content of redox-active compounds (i.e., antioxidants) in foods consumed in the United States. *American Journal of Clinical Nutrition* 84(1):95–135, 2006.

Step 4

1. Food and Nutrition Board, Institute of Medicine, National Academies. *Dietary Reference Intakes (DRIs): Estimated Average Requirements.* Available at www.iom.edu/Activities/Nutrition/SummaryDRIs/~/media/Files/Activity%20Files/Nutrition/DRIs/5_Summary%20Table%20Tables%201-4.pdf

Step 6

1. Kris-Etherton P, Eckel RH, Howard BV, St Jeor S et al. AHA Science Advisory: Lyon Diet Heart Study: Benefits of a Mediterranean-style, national cholesterol education program/American Heart Association Step I dietary pattern on cardiovascular disease. *Circulation* 103(13):1823–1825, 2001.

2. Sanders TA. DHA status of vegetarians. *Prostatglandins, Leukotrienes and Essential Fatty Acids* 81(2–3):137–141, 2009.
3. Conquer JA and Holub BJ. Supplementation with an algae source of docosahexaenoic acid increases (n-3) fatty acid status and alters selected risk factors for heart disease in vegetarian subjects. *Journal of Nutrition* 126(12):3032–3039, 1996.

Step 7

1. Weaver CM and Plawecki KL. Dietary calcium: adequacy of a vegetarian diet. *American Journal of Clinical Nutrition* 59(suppl):1238S–1241S, 1994.
2. Bolland MJ, Avenell A, Baron JA, Grey A et al. Effect of calcium supplements on risk of myocardial infarction and cardiovascular events: meta-analysis. *BMJ* 341:c3691, 2010. doi:10.1136/bmj.c3691.
3. Bolland MJ, Grey A, Avenell A, Gamble GD et al. Calcium supplements with or without vitamin D and risk of cardiovascular events: reanalysis of the Women's Health Initiative limited access dataset and meta-analysis. *BMJ* 342:d2040, 2011. doi:10.1136/bmj.d2040.

Index

Açai berries, 36
Africa, 3
algae blooms, 18
almond butter, 59
alpha-linolenic acid (ALA), 49, 58, 89, 90, 94–96
Alzheimer's disease, 9–10
amaranth, 47–48, 55
American Diabetes Association, 13
amino acids, 60, 67–68, 69, 72
angina, 12
animal foods
  animal proteins, 68
  elimination of, 126
  fisheries, 19–20
  and heart disease, 4
  inhumane treatment, 20–22
  livestock industry, 16–18
  and plant-based diet, 24–25
anthocyanins, 36
antibiotic resistance, 19
antioxidants, 7, 10, 14, 23, 33, 36
arthritis, 38
arugula, 26, 27, 28, 171
asthma, 38
atherosclerosis, 4
athletes, and protein, 69–72
ATP (adenosine triphosphate), 72
average life expectancy, 2
avocado, 58, 59

B vitamins, 23, 50, 54
  specific B vitamins
barley, 48, 55, 166
Barnard, Neal, 13
basmati rice, 47
beans, 40–45, 182–183
beet greens, 26, 27, 28, 102
berries, 36–37
beta-carotene, 33–34
beverages, 130
biodiversity, loss of, 19
black beans, 40, 41, 133, 205
blackberries, 36
blackstrap molasses, 131
blanching, 29
blood cholesterol. See cholesterol
blood oranges, 39
blood pressure, 12, 36
blood sugar, 47, 50
blueberries, 36
body mass index (BMI), 6
bok choy, 31, 32, 102
bone health, 27, 36, 98–100
braising, 29–30
bread, 45
breakfast, 65, 66, 70
breast cancer, 15, 16, 43, 47
bright orange vegetables, 33–34
broccoflower, 31
broccoli, 31, 32, 102, 195

broccoli raab. *See* rapini (broccoli raab)
broccoli sprouts, 31
broccolini, 31
brown rice, 48, 55
Brussels sprouts, 31, 32, 102, 200
buckwheat, 48, 55
bulgur, 52, 56
bycatch, 20

cabbage, 31, 32, 102, 173
caffeine, 100
calcium, 9, 15, 98–108, 115, 150
   bioavailable calcium, 102
   enhancing calcium absorption, 102
   food sources, 26, 28, 29, 31, 32, 38,
      41, 43, 47, 51, 101–104
   and healthy bones, 98–100
   recommended daily intake,
      100–101
   supplement, 104–107
   tips for getting more calcium,
      107–108
calcium carbonate, 105–106
calcium citrate, 105–106
calorie level, 150
calorie requirements, 67
cancer, 3, 7–8, 35, 36
   see also specific cancers
canned beans and lentils, 42
canola oil, 59, 136
carbohydrates, 74–86
   fibre, 76–79
   gluten, 84–85
   glycemic index, 80–84
   starches, 76
   sugars, 75
   tips for choosing healthy carbs,
      85–86
   and weight gain, 79–80
carbon dioxide emissions, 17
cardiovascular disease, 3–5
carrots, 33, 34, 198
cataracts, 27, 35, 38

cauliflower, 31, 32, 102, 196
celiac disease, 48, 84
chia seeds, 58, 59
chickpeas, 40, 133, 175, 179, 207
China, 3
Chinese grapefruit. *See* pomelos
cholesterol, 12, 14, 33, 36, 50, 87–88,
   89, 91–92
chronic diseases, 3
   see also health; specific diseases
citrus fruit, 38–40
Cleveland Clinic's Wellness Institute, 12
climate change, 17
coconut oil, 88
cognitive impairment, 38
cold pressed oils, 58
collard greens, 26, 27, 28, 102
colon cancer, 16, 47
complementary proteins, 68
complete proteins, 68
condiments, 128
convenience, 128
cooking methods
   beans and lentils, 42–43
   bright orange vegetables, 34
   cruciferous vegetables, 32
   leafy greens, 29–31
   whole grains, 54–57
copper, 47, 48, 50
corn, 45
coronary heart disease, 3–5, 12, 14
cracked wheat, 52
cranberries, 36
creatine supplements, 72
cruciferous vegetables, 31–33
cruelty to animals, 20–22
cyanocobalamin, 110

dandelion greens, 26, 27, 28
dementia, 9–10
desserts (recipes), 212–216
   Apple Raspberry Crisp with Maple
      Oat Topping, 212

Chocolate Fruit Fondue, 213
Cinnamon Pecan Baked Apples, 214
Fresh Berries with Chocolate and
    Toasted Coconut, 215
Tropical Fruit Salad with Lemon
    Maple Glaze, 216
DHA (docosahexaenoic acid), 91, 95,
    96–97
diabetes, 3, 5–6, 13, 35
    see also type 2 diabetes
Diet for a Small Planet (Lappé), 67
dinner, 66, 71
diverticulitis, 36
dried fruit, 131–132

edamame, 41, 42, 44, 132, 208, 211
egg replacements, 130
elemental calcium, 105
ellagic acid, 36
emmer (farro), 48–49
environmental protection, 16–20
enzymes, 54, 60
EPA (eicosapentaenoic acid), 91, 95,
    97
Esselstyn, Caldwell B. Jr., 12, 92
essential amino acids, 67–68
essential fatty acids, 89–91
estrogen, 15, 43
extra virgin olive oil, 136
eye health, 27

factory farms, 18
farmed fish, 19–20
farro, 48–49
fasting blood sugar, 12
fats. *See* healthy fats and oils
fibre, 23, 26, 31, 34, 38, 39, 41, 43, 46,
    47, 48, 49, 50, 54, 76–79, 85
fisheries, 19–20
flatulence, 78–79
flavonoids, 36, 38
flaxseed, 15, 49, 58, 59, 85
flaxseed oil, 136

folate, 26, 27–28, 29, 31, 32, 34, 38,
    39, 41, 43, 46, 47
food groups
    fruit, 34–40
    healthy fats and oils, 58–59
    key nutrients, 142
    legumes and soy, 40–45
    serving sizes, 142–148
    vegetables, 25–34
    whole grains, 45–57
free radicals, 14–15, 33
fruit, 34–40, 85
    berries, 36–37
    citrus fruit, 38–40
    dried fruit, 131–132
    glycemic index, selected fruits, 82
    iron content, 118–119
    key nutrients, 142
    one fruit serving, 34
    protein content, 64
    serving sizes, 146
    tips to increase fruit intake, 35

garbanzo beans, 41
gas, 78–79
George Washington University
    School of Medicine and Health
    Sciences, 13
glucagon, 60
glucosinolates, 31, 32
gluten, 84–85
gluten intolerance, 48, 84
glycemic index, 16, 47, 80–84
glycemic load, 83–84
goiter, 43, 44
grains. *See* whole grains
grapefruit, 38, 39
greenhouse gases (GHGs), 17, 19

HDL (good) cholesterol, 12, 88, 89
health
    specific diseases
        Alzheimer's disease, 9–10

bone health, 98–100
cancer, 3, 7–8, 35, 36
cardiovascular disease, 3–5
chronic diseases, 3
diabetes, 3, 5–6, 13, 35
eye health, 27
heart disease, 12, 14, 35, 41
metabolic syndrome, 11–12
obesity, 6–7
osteoporosis, 8–9
and plant-based diet, 2–10, 11–16
preventing illness, 10
stroke, 35
healthy fats and oils, 58–59, 87–97
ideal fat intake, 92–94
key nutrients, 142
low fat diet, 92
moderate fat diet, 92–93
omega-3 fats, 94–97
for the pantry, 136
requirements, 87
serving sizes, 148
tips for choosing the right fats, 97
types of fats, 87–92
heart disease, 3–5, 12, 14, 35, 41,
   106–107
hemp seeds, 58
herbs, 132
high blood pressure, 12
high-fructose corn syrup, 75
hip fractures, 8, 27
hummus, 132–133

impaired fasting glucose, 5
incomplete proteins, 68
India, 3
indoles, 31
inflammation, 15
insoluble fibre, 46, 77
instant oats, 50
insulin, 13, 14, 47, 60
intensive livestock operations (ILOs),
   16, 19, 20–22

iodine, 44–45, 151
iron, 28, 29, 41, 47, 50, 51, 53,
   116–120
isoflavones, 15, 43
isothiocyanates, 31, 32
isothy, 33

Japan, 3

kale, 26, 27, 28, 102, 203, 206
kamut, 49, 54, 56
kasha, 168
kidney beans, 40, 41, 102, 133

labels, 53–54
lacto-ovo vegetarians, 24
lacto-vegetarians, 24
land degradation, 17–18
Lappé, Frances Moore, 67
LDL (bad) cholesterol, 33, 87–88, 91
leaf lettuce, 26, 27, 28
leafy greens, 26–31, 51, 102
cooking, 29–31
nutrients in, 27–28
legumes, 40–45, 68, 127, 133
calcium content, 103
gluten-free diet, 85
glycemic index, 82
iron, 117
key nutrients, 142
protein content, 63
serving sizes, 143–144
zinc, 121
lemons, 38
lentils, 40–41, 41, 42, 85, 133, 167,
   180–181, 184
life expectancy, 2
lignans, 15, 46, 47, 49
lima beans, 41
limes, 38
linoleic acid, 89, 90, 91, 93–94
livestock industry, 16–18
low glycemic diet, 16, 47, 80–84

lunch, 65, 66, 70
lung cancer, 26
lutein, 27
lycopene, 38
Lyon Diet Heart Study, 93

macular degeneration, 27, 35, 38
magnesium, 15, 23, 28, 38, 41, 46, 47,
    48, 49
main courses (recipes), 175–193
    Balsamic Glazed Mushroom and Soy
        Burgers, 185–186
    Chickpea Curry, 175
    Chipotle Chili, 176
    Falafel Wrap with Lemon Tahini
        Sauce, 177–178
    Grilled Tofu with Sautéed Greens,
        187–188
    Moroccan Chickpea Stew, 179
    Mushroom Lentil Patties, 180–181
    Quinoa Stuffed Red Bell Peppers,
        193
    Sesame Crusted Tofu, 189
    Spicy Baked Tofu, 190
    Tempeh Vegetable Summer Rolls,
        191–192
    Three Bean Garden Chili, 182–183
    Whole-Grain Lentil Casserole,
        184
Mandarin oranges, 40
manganese, 47, 48
mass production, 3
meal plans, 149–153
    calorie level, 150
    moving food servings between
        meals, 153
    nutrient needs, 150–151
    7-day menu plan, 154–161
    using the meal plans, 151–152
meat analogues, 133
meat substitutes, 129
Mediterranean-style diet, 93–94
metabolic syndrome, 11

Meyer lemons, 40
microwaving, 31, 32
milks, non-dairy, 134
millet, 45, 49–50, 56
minerals, 15–16, 115–123
    see also specific minerals
Minneola tangelos, 39
miso, 133–134
modification of meals, 126–127
monounsaturated fats, 89
multivitamin and mineral supplement,
    151
mushrooms, 134, 180–181, 185–186,
    197
mustard greens, 26, 27, 28
myrosinase, 32

navel oranges, 38
navy beans, 41
niacin, 48
night blindness, 33
non-dairy milks, 134
non-essential amino acids, 67
nut butters, 58, 103, 135, 148
nutrient intake, 109–124
nutrient needs, 150–151
nutrition, and Canadians, 2
nutritional yeast, 135–136
nuts, 58, 63, 68, 102, 103, 117, 122,
    134–135, 148

oat bran, 50–51
oat flour, 51
oats, 45, 50–51, 56
obesity, 3, 6–7, 8, 75
obesogenic environment, 6–7
oils. See healthy fats and oils
olive oil, 59
olives, 58
omega-3 fatty acids, 89–91, 94–97,
    151
omega-6 fatty acids, 89–91, 95
oranges, 38, 39

Ornish, Dean, 92
osteoporosis, 8–9
ovarian cancer, 26
overfishing, 20
oxalates, 29, 102
oxidative stress, 15

pantry foods, 131–139
pasta, 45
pesco-vegetarians, 24
phenolic acids, 36
phosphoric acid, 100
phosphorus, 48
Physicians Committee for Responsible
    Medicine, 13
phytochemicals, 7, 14–15, 36, 42–43,
    46, 47
    see also specific phytochemicals
phytosterols, 46, 47
pinto beans, 40, 41, 102, 133
plant-based pantry, 131–139
Plant-Based Power Diet
    animal foods, 24–25
    and diabetes, 13
    environmental protection, 16–20
    food groups. *See* food groups
    and health, 2–10, 11–16
    and heart disease, 12
    kinder to animals, 20–22
    meal plans. *See* meal plans
    phytochemicals, 14–15
    preventing illness, 10
    protein, 62–67
    reasons to adopt diet, 11–22
    recipes. *See* desserts (recipes); main
        courses (recipes); recipes; salads
        (recipes); snacks (recipes);
        vegetable sides (recipes)
    serving sizes, 142–148
    transition to, 125–130
    vs. vegetarian diet, 20–21
    whole foods, plant-based diet, 23
polyunsaturated fats, 89–91

pomelos, 38, 40
potassium, 15, 26, 28, 31, 32, 34, 38,
    39, 41, 53
pre-diabetes, 5
processed grains, 47
prostate cancer, 38, 41
protein, 41, 43, 49, 53, 54, 60–73
    athletes, 69–72
    and calcium, 99
    combining proteins, 67–69
    in plant-based diet, 62–67
    recommended daily intakes,
        61–62
    tips for meeting protein needs, 73
    vital protein, 60–61
protein supplements, 71
pumpkin, 34

quick-cooking oats, 50
quinoa, 45, 51, 56, 170, 193

rapini (broccoli raab), 26, 27, 28
raspberries, 36
recipes
    desserts, 212–216
    main courses, 175–193
    salads, 166–174
    snacks, 205–211
    vegetable sides, 194–204
resistant starch, 46, 52
restaurant choices, 129
retinal, 33
rhubarb, 102
riboflavin, 50
rice, 45
risk factors
    Alzheimer's disease, 9
    heart disease, 4
    osteoporosis, 8–9
    stroke, 4
    type 2 diabetes, 6
rolled oats, 50
romaine lettuce, 26, 27, 28

rutabaga, 31
rye, 51, 54, 57

salads (recipes), 166–174
  Barley Salad with Lemon, Capers
    and Black Olives, 166
  Easy Lentil Salad, 167
  Kasha, Walnut and Apple Salad with
    Fresh Mint, 168
  Mango Cashew Salad, 169
  Quinoa Tabbouleh, 170
  Red Grape, Arugula and Toasted
    Walnut Salad, 171
  Roasted Beet Salad, 172
  Sesame Coleslaw, 173
  Spinach Salad with Strawberries,
    Pine Nuts and Champagne
    Vinaigrette, 174
saturated fats, 87–88
sautéing, 30, 32, 34
seed butters, 58, 103
seeds, 58, 63, 68, 117, 122, 134–135,
  148
seitan, 136
selenium, 46, 47, 48, 49
semi-vegetarians, 24
serving sizes, 142–148
sesame oil, 136
Seven Countries Study, 93
7-day menu plan, 154–161
Seville oranges, 39
snacks, 65, 70, 71, 129
snacks (recipes), 205–211
  Black Bean Hummus, 205
  Kale Chips with Sea Salt, 206
  Lemon Hummus, 207
  Sesame Ginger Edamame, 208
  Spicy Candied Walnuts, 209
  Tamari Roasted Almonds, 210
  Zesty Edamame, 211
sodium, 99–100
soluble fibre, 46, 49, 50, 77
soy beverages, 44

soy flour, 44
soy foods, 42–45, 63, 82, 103, 142,
  143–144
soy nuts, 44
soybeans, 40, 41, 42, 44, 133
spelt, 51–52, 54, 57
spices, 132
spinach, 26, 27, 28, 51, 102, 174, 202,
  204
split peas, 40
sprouted grains, 54
starches, 76
starchy vegetables, 57, 142, 145
steaming, 30–31, 32, 34
steel-cut oats, 50, 56
stir-frying, 32
stomach cancer, 26
strawberries, 36
stroke, 3–5, 35
sugars, 36, 75, 83
sulforaphane, 31
sweet potato, 33, 34
Swiss chard, 26, 28, 51, 102, 194,
  199

tahini, 136–137
tamoxifen, 43
tangerines, 38, 39, 40
teff, 52
tempeh, 42, 44, 137, 191–192
texturized vegetable protein (TVP),
  137
thiamin, 32, 38, 50
thyroid health, 43–44
tofu, 42, 44, 137–138, 187–188, 189,
  190
trans fats, 88–89
transition to plant-based diet,
  125–130
triglycerides, 12
tropical oils, 88
turnip, 31, 102
turnip greens, 26, 28, 102

type 2 diabetes, 3, 5–6, 11, 13, 16, 35, 41, 47
  see also diabetes

unsaturated fats, 89–91

Valencia oranges, 38–39
variety, 109, 150
vegans, 24
vegetable broth, 138
vegetable sides (recipes), 194–204
  Balsamic Swiss Chard, 194
  Broccoli with Sesame Dressing, 195
  Garlic Roasted Cauliflower, 196
  Grilled Balsamic Portobello
    Mushrooms, 197
  Lemon Swiss Chard, 199
  Maple Dijon Carrots, 198
  Oven Roasted Brussels Sprouts, 200
  Roasted Ginger Squash, 201
  Simple Sautéed Spinach with
    Lemon, 202
  Spicy Sautéed Kale, 203
  Spinach with Spicy Peanut Sauce,
    204
vegetables, 25–34, 85
  bright orange vegetables, 33–34
  calcium content, 104
  cruciferous vegetables, 31–33
  iron content, 118–119
  key nutrients, 142
  leafy greens, 26–31
  one vegetable serving, 25
  protein content, 64
  serving sizes, 147
  starchy vegetables, 57, 142, 145
  tips to increase vegetable intake, 26
vegetarian cookbooks, 127
vegetarian diet, 20–21
vinegars, 138
vitamin A, 26, 27–28, 31, 32, 33, 38
vitamin B₁. See thiamin

vitamin B₂. See riboflavin
vitamin B₆, 48
vitamin B₁₂, 72, 109–112, 150
vitamin C, 26, 27–28, 29, 31, 32, 34, 38, 39, 54
vitamin D, 9, 91, 102, 107, 112–114, 150–151
vitamin E, 23, 46, 47, 49, 50
vitamin K, 26, 27–28
vitamins, 15–16, 109–115
  see also specific vitamins

waist circumference, 12
walnut oil, 59, 136
water use and pollution, 18
weight loss, 36
Western diet, 3
wheat berries, 52, 54, 57
wheat bran, 85
white bread, 23
white semolina pasta, 47
whole foods, plant-based diet, 23
whole grains, 45–57, 63–64, 76
  cooking, 54–57
  glycemic index, selected whole
    grains, 81–82
  iron content, 118
  key nutrients, 142
  other whole-grain products, 53–54
  for the pantry, 138–139
  serving sizes, 144–145
  sprouted grains, 54
  types of, 47–53
  zinc, 122
whole wheat, 52
wild rice, 52–53, 57
winter squash, 33, 34, 201
worldwide obesity, 3

zeaxanthin, 27
zinc, 49, 53, 120–123